Strength Training at Home for Women Over 50

30-minute Workout Plans To Keep You Fit And Healthy

NJ's Fitsquad

NJ's Fitsquad Publication
2024

CONTENTS

INTRODUCTION

Imagine waking up each morning with renewed vitality, feeling stronger and more capable than ever. It's not just a dream—it's a reality within your reach. I want to challenge that notion in a world that often tells us that aging means slowing down. Let me share a story that might resonate with you.

Meet Susan, a vibrant woman in her mid-50s. Like many of us, Susan believed her strength would naturally diminish as she aged. Then she discovered something remarkable: through consistent strength training, she regained muscle and a newfound independence and zest for life. Susan's story is just one example of the countless women who have defied the stereotypes of aging through the power of strength training.

Studies show that women over 50 who engage in regular strength training experience profound benefits that defy common misconceptions about aging and exercise. Did you know that strength training can reverse the decline in muscle mass typically occurring with age? It's a game-changer, challenging the idea that getting older means becoming weaker.

As we face the unique challenges of life beyond 50, I understand the concerns and struggles you may face. Loss of muscle mass, decreasing bone density, and a metabolism that seems to slow each year— common pain points. However, what if I told you that strength training can turn these challenges into triumphs?

The goal of this book is simple yet transformative. I'm excited to offer ready-made exercise programs designed specifically for you—routines that take just 30 minutes daily, four days a week. That's right, only two hours a week for potentially life-changing results.

Perhaps a moment of realization about your body's changing needs led you here—the desire to maintain functional fitness, boost metabolism, or feel more confident and capable. Whatever your catalyst, know this book is tailored to meet you where you are.

Maybe you've noticed a decline in your overall strength and flexibility or are concerned about your joint health and injury prevention. Body image issues may have crept in, affecting your confidence levels. These catalysts, common among women over 50, are precisely why this book exists—to address your specific needs and empower you to take charge of your health and well-being.

Whether you've never worked out before, have tried but aren't sure where to start, or want to resume your fitness journey after a long break, this book is for you. The first two months of the workout program require minimal equipment—just a Chair, a mat, and two water bottles. As you progress, it will be beneficial to invest in some basic home workout equipment to continue your journey.

You'll encounter inspiring stories of women over 50 who have embraced strength training and transformed their lives. Their journeys illustrate the impact this approach can have.

Take Margaret, for example. At 58, she had never lifted weights in her life. However, she started a simple strength training routine at home. Within a few months, she was amazed at her increased energy levels and how her clothes fit better. Most importantly, she felt empowered and capable in her daily activities.

You'll gain more than knowledge—a roadmap to a better life. You'll find detailed exercise routines, safety precautions, nutritional guidance, and ways to monitor your progress. Whether you've never set foot in a gym or not, this is sure to be a wonderful guide. Compiling this book took many years of hands-on experience. I hope this will be a priceless resource for you.

Before starting any exercise program, it's vital to consult your healthcare provider to make sure it's safe for you to begin. Even after getting the go-ahead, stay mindful of warning signs like joint pain, swelling, heart palpitations, dizziness, or Chest pain. Your health and safety are so important as you embark on this journey.

Picture this: a life where you move easily and feel solid and capable in every endeavor. That's the result awaiting you. Imagine being able to lift groceries effortlessly, play with your grandchildren without worry, and confidently pursue new adventures.

In the words of Eleanor Roosevelt,

"You must do the thing you think you cannot do."

Let this book be your companion as you explore this empowering strength training and wellness path. Here's to embracing our strength at any age.

Let's dive in and begin this empowering process together.

CHAPTER ONE
Mindset For Fitness After 50

This caught my attention as somewhat interesting: When I asked ten seniors what their number-one New Year's resolution was this year, eight out of 10 people replied, "Make fitness part of my life and lead a well-balanced life." It's another matter entirely how many of these individuals truly follow through on their New Year's resolutions.

However, getting in shape is not a particularly tough resolution. If you put your mind in goal mode, exercising will come easily to you.

As we age, the fundamentals of healthy living—eating well, exercising regularly, getting enough sleep, and abstaining from harmful habits like smoking and binge drinking—become even more important. However, a new study indicates that a mindset toward aging may also play a significant role in determining how long we live and how well we feel as we age. It appears that having a positive mindset increases our likelihood of aging healthily.

Mindset And How It Affects Our Health

Embracing a positive outlook on aging can significantly enhance your quality of life. Studies have shown that individuals who maintain a cheerful attitude as they grow older tend to live longer, healthier lives.

They enjoy lower risks of chronic illnesses such as diabetes, stroke, and heart disease, allowing them to fully savor their golden years.

Those who have a different mindset about getting older typically suffer the consequences. They have an increased risk of diabetes, stroke, and heart disease while they are still living. Individuals who have a positive mindset on aging also perform better cognitively.

Researchers found that those who were satisfied with their aging and had positive attitudes about it were also more inclined to follow healthy routines. Individuals who believed that their aging would inevitably result in ill health, for example, were less likely to exercise.

Even if having a positive mindset doesn't always translate into making healthier decisions, it still has an impact. In a four-year study, individuals who felt content with their aging experience at the start of the study were less likely to suffer from depression, loneliness, or mobility difficulties than those who had internalized negative beliefs about aging.

Also, you must be ready with the mindset of doing the exercises repeatedly. It might get boring to do the same exercises, but that's what will bring you results. You will see results when you follow a particular program for at least 4 weeks continuously before moving on to a next one. Doing different exercises every day will confuse the muscles; however, shocking the muscles every 4 weeks will help you build them better.

Shifting Perspectives On Aging And Exercise

Everyone has a different perspective on aging. The thought of aging scares some people, and some greet it with naive ferocity! Your mindset matters more than you may realize. It has a significant impact on the standard of living you enjoy in your golden years.

The key to happy aging is mindset. It alludes to the notion that you will feel good about yourself, be physically active, and continue to fully engage in all aspects of life if you keep an optimistic view throughout your senior years, along with healthy habits, social interaction, and mental stimulation!

Although it may seem challenging, incorporating good aging practices into your everyday routine is actually rather simple.

Now that you understand the significance of positive aging, let's discuss five easy ways to change your perspective and include positivity in your daily life!

1. Embrace Your Age!

Age is just a number. You can understand that getting older is a natural part of life, one that everyone is trying to navigate, by keeping a youthful outlook and adjusting to your changing abilities.

Acknowledging and collaborating with the aging process is the first step towards unlocking the potential of positive aging. This makes it easier to handle the difficulties this stage of life brings, and instead, begin to look forward to the opportunities!

2. Give fitness a top priority!

Exercising for thirty minutes a day can completely transform your health. It can make you feel and look younger, make tasks go more smoothly, and reduce the risk of accidents and falls—all of which are necessary for keeping a positive attitude.

However, before you go out on this empowering adventure, bear in mind these three fundamental thoughts:

Believe in Yourself

First and foremost, believe in yourself. It's common to have doubts or fears, especially if strength training is new to you. Remember, you are capable and resilient. Strength training is not just for the young; it's incredibly beneficial at any age. It can improve your muscle mass, balance, bone density, and overall quality of life. Embrace the mindset that you can do this. Each step you take, no matter how small, is a step towards a stronger, healthier you. Believe in your ability to grow stronger and more capable each day.

Have Patience

Patience is essential. Results in strength training or any other physical activity don't happen overnight, especially when you're starting later in life. Understand that progress might be slower, and that's perfectly okay. The journey itself is valuable, teaching you about your body, your limits, and your potential. Celebrate small victories along the way—being consistent or lifting a little heavier, feeling more energetic, or simply mastering a new exercise. Patience will help you stay motivated and keep you from getting discouraged when the progress seems slow. Remember, it's not about instant results but about sustainable, long-term health benefits.

Consistency is the Key (Discipline)

Consistency is paramount. Discipline in your routine will yield the best results over time. Make strength training a regular part of your life. This doesn't mean you have to spend hours in the gym; even short, regular sessions can make a significant difference. Create a routine that suits your way of life and stick to it. Consistency helps your body adapt and grow stronger.

Moreover, it builds a habit, making exercise a natural part of your routine rather than a chore. On days when motivation wanes, rely on your discipline to keep you going. Remember, showing up consistently is more important than having the perfect workout every time.

Starting strength training above 50 is a bold and wonderful choice. Believe in yourself, be patient with your progress, and stay consistent in your efforts. These principles will not only help you achieve your fitness goals but also empower you with greater confidence and vitality in your daily life. Embrace this journey with enthusiasm and determination—you have the strength within you to achieve great things!

Remember, regular strength training goes beyond physical benefits. It also promotes mental well-being, reduces stress, and enhances abilities like problem-solving, resilience, decision-making, reasoning, and focus. This holistic improvement in both body and mind will enrich every aspect of your life, making you feel more empowered, capable, and vibrant each day.

3. Stay Connected!

A good aging plan also includes establishing and preserving close relationships. By doing this, you can fight loneliness, boost your confidence, and create a feeling of community. Not sure where to start? Try any of the following to meet new people or rekindle old friendships:

- Join a social group, such as a reading club, pickleball league, birding club, or volunteer group.
- Plan a monthly potluck with friends or family, where each person brings a different dish.
- Make it a point to support your grandchildren (if you have one) by going to their sporting events and performances; they will appreciate your presence!

4. Nurture Healthy Habits!

Eating a balanced diet is most important to the aging process. Eating healthfully promotes heart health and helps you maintain a healthy weight. Follow these easy guidelines to help you Stick to your diet:

- Include lean proteins, lots of veggies (particularly orange, red, and green ones), whole grain substitutions when possible, and low-fat dairy products.
- Avoid sugar-filled beverages and drink plenty of water.
- Age-related deficiencies in vitamin D and fiber should be sought out in meal selections.
- To keep performing at your best, there are other habits you should give up. First, get enough sleep. The body needs a good night's sleep to function well. Abstain from smoking and heavy alcohol use. Both have the potential to harm people of all ages seriously.

5. Develop Mental Agility!

Similar to your body, your mind grows when you challenge it. A strong mind keeps you focused and is essential to your positive aging formula. To give your brain the activity it requires, incorporate games like Sudoku and crossword puzzles into your everyday routine.

Acquiring a new skill can also enhance intelligence. See whether any nearby institutions, such as a community center or university, provide any engaging classes for developing your skills. Acquiring a new skill fosters a positive mindset and increases self-confidence. Not to add, it's enjoyable and gives you something to look forward to!

Setting And Achieving Realistic Fitness Goals

Did you know that forming a healthy habit takes an average of 66 days? This is based on research published in the European Journal of Social Psychology. Researchers discovered that if adults set small, attainable goals and stick with them for a few months, the habit will gradually become nearly second nature to them, much like brushing your teeth before bed or putting lotion on after a bath.

Perhaps you've recently dealt with a significant medical problem, and your goal is to recover as soon as possible. Maybe you'd like to improve your lifestyle because you're concerned about your physical health and feel like you need to exercise more.

But how are such goals set? How can you set up your schedule to accommodate a new, healthful habit? There is actually a trick to setting and accomplishing goals. Let's examine this.

Before You Begin

Remember to discuss your goals with your doctor before making any adjustments to your regular daily health routine. A new diet, an exercise regimen, or a supplement that seems promising might not be the best fit for you, and you may have any underlying medical concerns. Your physician can advise you on its viability and may even recommend better options than what you had in mind.

Additionally, having a medical alert system with fall detection on hand is a smart idea for women over 50. This helps you sustain an active lifestyle and protects you around the clock, with assistance available whenever you need it. A fall alert can literally save your life if you have an emergency, such as a fall, and you need to contact for help right away. It's simple and quick to call help when you have an alert button at your fingertips.

Let's get started with realistic goal-setting now.

How Do SMART Goals Work?

A business concept can occasionally be brilliantly adapted for a personal plan. The acronym SMART is one that many executives in business are familiar with. SMART is a good technique to set a goal and measure your progress toward it. Here's what it means when modified to represent personal growth:

S: Specific and Simple

This means your goal must be as specific as possible. For example, instead of a goal to run a mile in one minute, you can set a specific goal to run a shorter distance, going faster each time until you reach the "wall" and are unable to go any quicker; at that point, your goal can change.

M: Measurable and Maintainable

This means that your goal must have clear criteria for tracking progress and determining when it has been achieved. For example, instead of a goal to "improve cardiovascular health," you can set a measurable goal to "walk an extra mile every day."

A: Achievable and Age-Appropriate

It's crucial to confirm that this goal is suitable for your age. This entails examining your strengths and weaknesses with objectivity. Even while kickboxing appears like a great way to get in shape—which it is—is that something your body is capable of achieving? Put differently, pick goals that align with your current stage of life.

R: Relevant and Realistic

Your goal must be something that makes sense for your life. It could be a goal to increase your mobility. It could be an attempt to reach a specific body weight on the scale. Alternatively, it could be as easy as deciding to always take your prescription on schedule.

T: Timely and Tailored

The goal you choose is a way to move you into a healthier, happier future. Because of your aging body, it is important to know that it takes time to show results. Examine your current situation in life and consider what adjustments would help you improve it.

Success Stories: Real-Life Inspirations

Here are inspiring stories of real women over fifty who transformed their lives through strength training, proving that it's never too late to start and thrive.

Jane's Journey to Strength

Jane Fonda, the iconic actress and fitness guru, had always been an advocate for staying active, but it wasn't until she turned 55 that she discovered the true power of strength training. After years of focusing on aerobic exercise, she decided to incorporate weight lifting into her routine to maintain her bone density and muscle mass. The results were astounding. Not only did she feel stronger physically, but her mental clarity and energy levels soared. Jane's commitment to strength training transformed her life, proving that it's never too late to start and thrive. She became an inspiration to women everywhere, showing that age is just a number when it comes to achieving new health milestones.

Oprah's Empowerment through Exercise

Oprah Winfrey, known for her incredible journey of self-improvement, took a significant step in her fitness regimen at the age of 60 by embracing strength training. Struggling with weight and health issues for years, Oprah found that lifting weights brought a new level of empowerment and resilience. The strength training not only sculpted her body but also enhanced her mental fortitude. She noticed improvements in her problem-solving skills, decision-making abilities, and overall stress levels. Oprah's transformation underscored her message of self-care and perseverance, encouraging women over fifty to take control of their health and well-being through the powerful benefits of strength training.

Celebrating Your Progress And Adjusting Goals

Recognizing and celebrating your progress, no matter how small, is crucial to your fitness journey. Each step forward, whether it's lifting a slightly heavier weight, feeling more energetic, or mastering a new exercise, is a victory. These small milestones are the building blocks of your long-term success. By acknowledging these achievements, you fuel your motivation and keep a positive mindset.

Life is full of unexpected events and challenges. There will be times when your fitness routine might need to take a back seat due to family commitments, health issues, or other priorities. It's important to understand that adjusting your goals during these times is not a step back. It's a realistic and compassionate approach to maintaining balance in your life. Flexibility in your fitness journey is key. Remember, it's okay to take breaks and adjust your goals. This doesn't diminish your progress or commitment.

When you're ready, you can always return to a routine that includes fitness. The strength and resilience you've built are still there, and you can pick up where you left off or even start fresh with new goals. Your journey is unique, and every step you take, no matter how big or small, contributes to your overall well-being. Embrace the process, be kind to yourself, and keep moving forward. You have the power to thrive at any stage of life.

Interactive Reflection

What's the biggest barrier you face in starting or maintaining an exercise routine, and how can you address it this week?

Think about what holds you back—time constraints, lack of motivation, or perhaps uncertainty about where to start. Reflect on one actionable step you can take this week to overcome this barrier. Maybe it's setting aside 10 minutes a day for exercise, finding a workout buddy, or seeking out a fitness class that excites you.

What are one or two fitness goals you consider realistic and achievable within the next three months?

Set specific, measurable, and attainable goals. For example, it could be increasing your strength by lifting heavier weights, improving your stamina by walking longer distances or enhancing flexibility through regular stretching. Write down these goals and outline the steps you'll take to achieve them.

Which aspect of the success stories resonated with you the most, and how can it inspire your fitness journey?

Reflect on the stories of Jane Fonda and Oprah Winfrey. What elements of their journeys inspire you? Is it their resilience, their ability to overcome challenges or their dedication to self-improvement? Think about how their experiences can motivate you to take the next step in your fitness journey.

PERSONAL REFLECTION JOURNAL

Use this space to jot down your thoughts and feelings. Consider your personal experiences with aging and exercise, the mental health benefits you seek from staying active, and the inspiration you draw from the success stories shared. This journal is your space to reflect, plan, and track your journey.

Date: _____

Personal experiences with aging and exercise:

_____

_____

_____

Mental health benefits I seek from staying active:

_____

_____

_____

Inspiration drawn from success stories:

_____

_____

_____

SIMPLE, ACTIONABLE FITNESS PLAN

Creating a fitness plan doesn't have to be complicated. Here's a template to help you integrate fitness into your daily life.

1. Set Your Goals:

Short-term (next three months):

_____

_____

_____

Long-term (next year):

_____

_____

_____

2. Weekly Schedule:

Monday: Activity: _____ Duration _____

Tuesday: Activity: _____ Duration _____

Wednesday: Activity: _____ Duration _____

Thursday: Activity: _____ Duration _____

Friday: Activity: _____ Duration _____

Saturday: Activity: _____ Duration _____

Sunday: Activity: _____ Duration _____

3. Progress Tracking:

Weekly Check-In:

What went well this week?

_____

What challenges did I face?

_____

How can I adjust for next week?

_____

Remember, this plan is flexible. Adapt it to fit your lifestyle and needs. The goal is to create a sustainable, enjoyable fitness routine that enhances your well-being. You've got this!

After learning to have the right mindset, we're now turning our attention inward. In the next chapter, we'll navigate the physical shifts that come with age, understand how exercise can ease menopause symptoms, and learn the pivotal role of strength training for bone health. It's time to adjust our fitness routines to our body's evolving needs.

CHAPTER TWO
Understanding Your Changing Body

As you move through your 50s and beyond, you may notice subtle and not-so-subtle changes in your body. Perhaps you've felt a shift in your energy levels, noticed changes in your muscle tone, or experienced fluctuations in your weight. You might find that your joints feel stiffer or your balance isn't quite what it used to be. These changes can be frustrating and sometimes even discouraging, making you wonder if you can ever feel strong and vibrant again.

But here's the empowering truth: these changes are a natural part of aging and understanding them is the first step towards reclaiming your strength and vitality. This chapter is dedicated to helping you understand the "why" behind what you're experiencing. You can make informed decisions that enhance your health and well-being by gaining insight into how your body is evolving.

It's normal to feel a mix of emotions about these changes but remember, you've made the right decision by choosing to educate and empower yourself. By reading through this chapter and the ones that follow, you're taking steps toward living your best life. Together, we will explore these changes, leverage them to your advantage, and help you thrive in this new chapter of your life.

Physical Changes And Their Impacts

Maintaining an active lifestyle can help you look and feel younger, especially in your 50s when you may start to notice the first minor changes in your skin or metabolism.

What can you expect from this decade? Although every person ages differently and lifestyle plays a significant part, you will notice changes in your physical and emotional well-being that are both difficult to overlook and difficult to detect.

Read on to learn more about the natural physical changes that occur after fifty.

Bones

Your body replaces weaker bone cells with stronger ones while you're younger. You have more broken-down bone cells by the time you reach your 50s. This indicates that your bones deteriorate over time. Eat foods high in calcium and vitamin D to protect them. Exercises that include bearing weight and resistance, such as walking, hiking and weightlifting, can also help your bones stay strong.

Muscle

Beyond the age of 50, muscle mass begins to lose more quickly, and you may also become less physically strong. Lifting weights or performing strength training activities focusing on both upper and lower body muscles two to three times a week is the greatest approach to stopping this slide. You will increase your lean muscle mass and sharpen your sense of balance, both of which will be beneficial as you age.

Joints

You'll start to see the impacts of this thinning of the cartilage and tissue that cushion your joints in your 50s. (Men might get it earlier.) Start with your posture to prevent arthritis and joint pain. You put Pressure on your joints when you slouch. Additionally, monitor your weight because excess weight might strain your joints. Drink a lot of water as well. Your body takes fluid from joint tissue when you're thirsty.

Heart

The risk of having a heart attack increases after the age of fifty. Exercise can help maintain the health of your heart and blood vessels; try to get in at least 30 minutes each day. (Even quick strolls count.) Maintain normal blood Pressure and weight ranges. If you haven't quit smoking yet, this is the ideal moment. Cigarette smoking is one of the main causes of heart disease.

Hair

Hair can begin to recede and thin around the age of fifty. In addition, depending on your family history and ethnic group, it will most likely become gray. You can color your hair if you're self-conscious about how "old" it looks.

Hearing

A significant portion of the over-50 population—up to 40%—has hearing loss. In addition to aging naturally, some medical conditions, including diabetes, high blood Pressure, and heart problems, might eventually impact your hearing, as can your genes. Consult your doctor about a hearing test if you have any concerns. Individuals with poor hearing are more prone to isolate themselves from friends and family and experience depression.

Skin

Any sun damage you may have had as a carefree child will now show. You should keep an eye out for any indications of skin cancer and be aware of age spots. It's not too late to start protecting your skin if you didn't do so when you were younger. Use sunscreen with at least 30 SPF daily and get screened for skin cancer annually. Your skin will likely feel dryer and become irritated more readily. An odorless moisturizer (not lotion) can be helpful.

Vision

When reading on your phone, you may need to squint since, as you age, the lenses in your eyes become more rigid. They can't swiftly move from focusing on the distance to a close-up. You may be able to get by with over-the-counter glasses, or you may require a new prescription for vision correction. Your eyesight will change more as you age, so schedule regular examinations.

Health Screenings

While it is true that your chance of health problems increases as you get older, some tests can identify potential problems early on. Probably one of these will be a colonoscopy to look for colon cancer. Women should have annual mammograms and Pap smears every three years, and men should have screenings for testicular and prostate cancer every three years. Inform your doctor if there is a family history of the disease. They might also want you to undergo additional testing. More screenings include blood tests to check for diabetes and any other deficiencies.

Menopause

The average age at which a woman's menstruation ends is 51. During menopause, you may experience various symptoms affecting your daily life. Hot flashes can be intense, causing sudden feelings of warmth and sweating. You might also notice mood changes, such as irritability and depression, which are common during this transition. Dry skin and thinning hair are other physical changes you may encounter. Also, the vaginal lining can become drier and thinner, making sex uncomfortable. It's important to consult your physician for relief through treatments like hormone therapy and antidepressants. Simple lifestyle adjustments, such as using moisturizers for dry skin and ensuring enough sleep, can also help manage these symptoms.

The Role Of Strength Training In Managing Menopause Symptoms

It's possible that you've heard that strength training becomes more crucial as you age. However, why does it significantly impact your health and happiness both before and after menopause? Here, I'll discuss why including this kind of exercise in your routine can benefit your health in a number of ways.

What is strength training?

Strength training involves exercises that improve muscle endurance and strength. This indicates that resistance is present when your muscles contract. This could be a fitness band, weight, or step.

Strength training doesn't always include lifting weights or going to the gym. It can involve a variety of activities.

Some effective strength training includes:

- Hillwalking
- Climbing stairs
- Pilates
- Resistance band exercises
- HIIT workouts
- Cycling
- Bodyweight workouts

Additionally, you can build the strength of your muscles by utilizing kettlebells or dumbbells. Even simple tasks like carrying your shopping bag home or getting out of a Chair without using your arms might help you gain strength. So, even if you're not a big gym goer, you can still easily add strength training into your routine.

Why is strength training important for menopause?

Your hormones change during perimenopause. Menopausal symptoms like anxiety and hot flashes may result from this. However, your levels of estrogen—the female sex hormone—begin to fall permanently at the end of this period.

This has a variety of effects on your body. Osteoporosis, in particular, may become more likely as a result of estrogen reduction. This is because estrogen has a role in maintaining the strength of your bones. You run a greater risk of fractures and bone density loss when estrogen levels drop.

Strength training helps reduce this effect. Studies have shown that women who exercise daily can lower their risk of developing osteoporosis after menopause. Another study looked at women who already had postmenopausal osteoporosis. It discovered that women who engaged in twice-weekly strength training had higher bone density than those who did not.

In addition to maintaining strong bones and muscles after menopause, strength training can benefit you in the following ways.

Heart health

Following menopause, there may be a higher chance of cardiac problems. This is because estrogen also aids in heart disease prevention. You run a higher risk when you have less of it. Fortunately, strength training offers a beneficial and preventive impact on heart disease.

Menopausal women who regularly engaged in strength training had lower levels of inflammatory molecules associated with heart disease. Additionally, there is evidence to support the idea that resistance training lowers a person's chance of experiencing a heart attack or stroke. Thus, it makes sense to incorporate strength training into your daily routine.

Weight management

Unfortunately, weight gain may become more prevalent with menopause. Visceral fat, the dangerous fat that can accumulate around your internal organs, may rise as a result. The reduction of estrogen during menopause can be one of the unclear causes of these changes in body composition.

At this stage of life, strength exercise can help improve metabolism. Gaining muscular mass can raise your resting metabolic rate, which is advantageous since it means you burn more energy even when at rest. Therefore, building muscle will aid in weight management during and after menopause.

Mental well-being

In addition to the physical benefits, strength training is a popular choice for people's mental health. You can be more prone to mood fluctuations or elevated anxiety throughout the menopause. The variations in hormones are generally to blame for this.

Research indicates that strength exercise can enhance the mental well-being of menopausal women. This could be due to the production of feel-good hormones called endorphins, which may also help with sleep.

Adjusting Workout Routines To Your Body's Needs

Adjusting your fitness routine to match your body's evolving needs isn't just about changing exercises; it's about truly listening to your body, allowing for adequate rest, and recognizing when to push and pause.

As a woman over 50, your body's responses to exercise are different than they were in your younger years. You might notice that it takes longer to recover after a workout or that some exercises don't feel as comfortable as they once did. This is completely normal and part of the natural aging process.

Here's how to adjust your workout routine to ensure it's aligned with your body's needs:

Listen to Your Body

Pay close attention to how your body feels during and after exercise. If an exercise causes pain or discomfort, it might be time to modify it or choose a different one that achieves the same benefits without strain. Your body is incredibly wise, and tuning into its signals can help you avoid injury and maximize your results.

Allow for Adequate Rest

Rest is crucial for recovery, especially as you age. Muscles need time to repair and grow stronger after being challenged. Schedule rest days into your routine, and do not push yourself too hard. This doesn't mean you have to be inactive on rest days; gentle activities like walking or stretching can aid recovery and keep you moving.

Recognize When to Push and When to Pause

There will be days when you feel full of energy and ready to push your limits. Embrace those days and challenge yourself. However, there will also be days when your body feels tired or strained. On those days, it's important to pause and opt for a lighter workout or take a rest day. This balance helps prevent burnout and keeps you motivated in the long run.

Adjust Exercises for Your Needs

Modify exercises to suit your current fitness level and physical condition. For instance, if high-impact exercises like running or jumping are hard on your joints, switch to low-impact alternatives like swimming, cycling, or walking. Use lighter weights or resistance bands to build strength without overloading your muscles and joints.

Focus on Flexibility and Balance

Incorporate flexibility and balance exercises into your routine. These exercises can also help reduce fall risk and improve overall mobility.

Adjusting your workout routine is about honoring where you are in your fitness journey. It's not about doing less; it's about doing what's best for your body right now. By listening to your body, allowing for adequate rest, and recognizing when to push and when to pause, you're setting yourself up for long-term success and well-being. You're making a wise and powerful choice to stay active and healthy, and this journey is entirely yours to navigate with confidence and grace.

Five Essential Tools To Transform Yourself

To truly transform your health and fitness journey, having the right tools can make all the difference. Here are five essential items that can help you stay on track and achieve your goals:

1. Weighing Scale

A weighing scale is a fundamental tool in monitoring your progress. While it's important not to become obsessed with the numbers, regularly checking your weight can help you stay aware of your overall health trends. Remember, it's about losing weight and understanding how your body changes with muscle gain and fat loss. Use the scale as one of several indicators of your progress and celebrate non-scale victories like increased energy and improved strength or how well your old clothes may fit in.

2. Food Scale

A food scale is handy for managing portions and understanding nutritional intake. As you age, your metabolism changes, making it important to be mindful of what and how much you eat. Weighing your food can help you get the right amount of nutrients without overeating. It's a practical way to maintain a balanced diet and support your fitness goals, helping you feel more in control of your eating habits.

3. Water Bottle

Staying hydrated is essential for overall health, especially as you get older. Dehydration can affect everything from your energy levels to your skin health. Keeping a water bottle with you encourages regular hydration throughout the day. Aim for at least eight glasses of water daily, but remember that your needs might vary based on your activity level and the climate. A reusable water bottle is a convenient reminder to drink more water and care for your body.

4. Step Tracker

A step tracker, or pedometer, is a great way to monitor your daily activity levels. Regular movement is crucial for maintaining health and vitality, and setting a daily step goal can motivate you to stay active. Whether walking around the neighborhood or taking the stairs more often, tracking your steps helps ensure you incorporate enough physical activity into your routine. It's a simple yet powerful tool to keep you moving and motivated.

5. Calorie Tracker

A calorie tracker can be a helpful tool for managing your weight and understanding your eating habits. By logging what you eat, you can gain insights into your calorie intake and ensure you meet your nutritional needs without overindulging. Many apps such as "MyFitnessPal app" or "Cronometer" also provide information on macronutrients and vitamins, helping you make more informed choices about your diet. It's an effective way to stay accountable and adjust as needed to support your fitness goals.

Transforming your health and fitness journey over 50 requires the right mindset and the right tools. These tools are all valuable aids that can help you stay on track and make informed decisions about your health. Each tool serves a unique purpose, contributing to a holistic approach to your well-being. Embrace these tools, stay motivated, and remember that every small step you take brings you closer to your goals. You've got the power to transform yourself and thrive at any age!

Interactive Reflection

What physical change has been most noticeable for you, and how has it affected your daily life?

Think about the physical changes you've observed in your body recently. It might be changes in muscle tone, joint stiffness, weight fluctuations, or something else. Reflect on how these changes have impacted your daily activities, energy levels, and overall well-being. Use this space to write down your thoughts and insights.

Most noticeable physical change:

_____

_____

_____

Impact on daily life:

_____

_____

_____

MENOPAUSE SYMPTOMS JOURNAL

Understanding your body's patterns during menopause can help you manage symptoms more effectively. Use this journal to note down your symptoms over time. This can help you identify patterns, triggers, and effective strategies for relief.

Date: _____

Symptoms Experienced:

Hot Flashes: _____

Night Sweats: _____

Mood Swings: _____

Sleep Disturbances: _____

Fatigue: _____

Weight Gain: _____

Other Symptoms: _____

Notes:

Activities or foods that seemed to trigger symptoms:

_____

_____

_____

Strategies that helped alleviate symptoms:

_____

_____

_____

Overall feeling today:

_____

_____

_____

After understanding the changes that come with aging, you should next understand the importance of nutrition and daily habits. In the next chapter, we'll uncover how the foods we eat and our lifestyle choices can dramatically enhance the benefits of our physical activities, support our bodily changes, and elevate our overall quality of life.

CHAPTER THREE
Nutrition And Lifestyle

Imagine waking up daily feeling energized, vibrant, and confident in your body. Picture yourself enjoying meals that taste delicious and nourish you from the inside out. Envision living a lifestyle that supports your health, happiness, and longevity. This is not a distant dream—it's entirely within your reach.

As a woman over 50, your nutritional needs and lifestyle habits majorly affect how you look and feel. Your body undergoes changes that require adjustments in how you feel and care for yourself. Embracing these changes can lead to a transformative experience, improving your mental and physical well-being.

This chapter is your guide to making those impactful changes. By understanding the significance of healthy nutrition and adopting healthy lifestyle habits, you can attain a renewed sense of vitality. You'll discover practical tips, inspiring ideas, and actionable steps to help you look and feel your best.

You've made an excellent choice by choosing this book. Together, we'll explore the power of nutrition and lifestyle and how they can significantly enhance your quality of life. Get ready to begin on the path of self-discovery and transformation. Say "yes" to the changes that will make you look good and feel even better.

Essential Nutrients For Women Over 50

As you age, your body's nutritional needs increase, making it essential to focus on getting the right balance of nutrients to support your health and vitality.

From influencer-led weight loss initiatives to celebrity-endorsed eating plans, we are unable to avoid complex diets that promise amazing outcomes. Whether it's celery juice, cabbage soup, or intermittent fasting, most diet plans center on creating a calorie deficit to lead a healthy lifestyle.

However, the "calories in, calories out" philosophy is a little limiting because, in addition to individual differences in age, size, and form, there are also individual differences in activity levels.

So, if you're calorie counting and still not achieving your goals, perhaps it's time to rethink your method. TDEE and BMR are useful for that.

Firstly, let's cover the basics: What is a 'calorie'? What is Metabolism? What are Macro and Micronutrients? What is a whole meal?

Calories are units of energy that fuel your body, while metabolism is the procedure by which your body transforms what you consume into energy.

Macro and micronutrients refer to the building blocks of your diet: macronutrients include proteins, fats, and carbohydrates, which provide energy and support bodily functions, while micronutrients, like vitamins and minerals, are needed in smaller amounts but are crucial for overall health.

A whole meal includes the right portions of both macronutrients and micronutrients. This balance ensures you're fueling your body effectively, promoting optimal health, and feeling your best.

For women over 50, this means paying extra attention to nutrient-dense foods that support bone health, muscle maintenance, and overall energy levels. By embracing the right mix of nutrients, you can navigate this new chapter with strength and vitality.

What Is BMR?

Basal Metabolic Rate is the number of calories your body burns at rest. In other words, these are the calories required by your body for sustenance.

Regardless of their level of physical activity, people use BMR and other indicators to calculate how many calories they burn each day. By accounting for your workouts and exercise, you can use BMR to determine the number of calories you consume daily to reach your weight loss goal.

Basal implies "forming or belonging to a bottom base or layer." It's the fundamentals. However, this does not mean there isn't activity below the surface. These processes burn 60–75% of your daily caloric intake.

While you lie in bed, consider everything happening: your lungs must draw in and expel oxygen, your heart must pump blood, and oxygen must reach your brain and other parts of your body.

The energy needed for essential functions like blood circulation, breathing, and temperature control varies according to height, weight, age, and gender.

Similar to but different from RMR (resting metabolic rate) and REE (resting energy expenditure), BMR is often used interchangeably with BEE (basal energy expenditure). Although many people misinterpret their definitions, BMR is a little more restrictive than RMR. Patients must stay overnight at a testing center the night before their formal test to calculate their true basal metabolic rate. You'll need an appointment if you'd like to be that precise.

That being said, making an appointment is not required!

The practical techniques for calculating BMR—which, when computed with a formula instead of testing, effectively becomes RMR—will be examined for our purposes.

It can be challenging to determine your exact basal metabolic rate, but nonetheless, you can calculate it using a formula to achieve your weight loss goal.

How to Calculate Your BMR

While there is disagreement over the most accurate way to compute BMR, all formulas have certain fundamental components:

- Age
- Gender
- Weight
- Activity
- Height
- Body Fat (optional)

The quickest method to determine your basal metabolic rate is to use an online calculator, which can be found at

https://www.calculator.net/bmr-calculator.html

Alternatively, if you'd rather handle the arithmetic yourself, you can utilize the gender-specific formulas known as the Harris-Benedict Formula.

Male BMR formula:

66 + (6.23 x weight) + (12.7 x height) - (6.8 x age)

For instance, if you weigh 170 pounds, are 5'11" tall, and are 43 years old, your BMR is 66 + (6.23 x 170) + (12.7 x 71) – (6.8 x 43) = 1,734.4 calories.

Female BMR formula:

655 + (4.35 x weight) + (4.7 x height) - (4.7 x age)

For instance, if you weigh 130 pounds, are 5'3" tall, and are 36 years old, your BMR is 665 + (4.35 x 130) + (4.7 x 63) – (4.7 x 36) = 1,357.4 calories.

Understood? Okay, let's go! After using a BMR calculator, your next step should be to look at TDEE.

WHAT IS TDEE?

Total Daily Energy Expenditure (TDEE) estimates daily caloric expenditure, including physical exercise. It is calculated by multiplying your BMR by 1.2 to 1.9, depending on your activity level.

TDEE is just BMR with additional estimations. The only difference in the algorithm is that a multiplier based on your daily activity level is included.

For example, your BMR would be multiplied by 1.55 if you worked out three to five days a week.

To calculate TDEE, think of it as adding everything you do in a typical day to your basal metabolic rate. If you start using a TDEE calculator, you will probably lose weight.

This covers every physical activity we engage in and all the small daily tasks we complete, such as taking a shower, strolling about the workplace, taking out the trash, petting the dogs, and yelling at the television. You know—just normal stuff.

Simply put, your TDEE is your BMR plus the total number of calories required to perform your daily activities. If your calorie intake and TDEE are equal, you will stay at your current weight.

You will shed pounds and show more lean body mass if your calorie intake is lower than your TDEE. It really is that easy.

Calculating Your TDEE

Use these multiples based on how much you exercise:

- Your BMR should be multiplied by 1.2 if you rarely exercise
- Your BMR should be multiplied by 1.55 if you exercise one to three days a week
- Your BMR should be multiplied by 1.375 if you exercise three to five days a week

- Your BMR should be multiplied by 1.725 if you exercise six to seven days a week
- Multiply your BMR by 1.9 if you work out twice daily and have a physical job.

Like basal metabolic rate, you can use the TDEE formula online calculator at: https://www.calculator.net/tdee-calculator.html to quickly determine your total daily energy expenditure.

So, assuming a man works out three days a week, he needs 1,734.4 x 1.55, or 2,688.3 calories per day.

Also, the woman in the case needs 1,357.4 x 1.725 = 2,342.5 calories per day if she works out six days a week. You can start by reducing 300 to 500 calories; for example, if TDEE is 2342.5 calories per day, you can start at 1900/2000 calories per day to see weight loss and increase to 2600 calories per day to see weight gain.

Fiber And Protein: Your Best Allies

You must pay close attention to your food to age well and maintain your health. Eating more fruits and vegetables is recommended to increase the intake of vital vitamins and minerals. However, fiber and protein are also crucial components of a healthy diet. What are the recommendations for seniors' protein and fiber intake?

Protein is crucial to a healthy diet because it provides the amino acids required to sustain body structure. Put differently, we need protein in our diets to compensate for what we lose.

Fruits and veggies are highly recommended because of their vitamin, mineral, and fiber content. The latter benefits have been shown to prevent colon cancer, diabetes, obesity, cholesterol, and related disorders. For women above 50, fiber intake should be provided through a varied diet.

Including fiber and protein in every meal is a powerful way to enhance your health, especially as a woman over 50. Fiber in fruits, vegetables, whole grains, and legumes aids digestion by promoting regular bowel movements and preventing constipation, which can become more common with age. It also helps regulate blood sugar and lowers cholesterol, contributing to heart health.

On the other hand, protein is necessary to preserve muscle mass, which declines with age. Protein-rich foods include fish, eggs, dairy, lean meats, beans, and nuts. Protein and fiber also promote a feeling of fullness, helping you manage your weight and reduce cravings.

Sample Nutritious Recipes For Everyday Eating

1. Brown bread toast sandwich

The brown bread toast sandwich combines fresh vegetables, providing a balanced, nutrient-dense meal perfect for digestion and overall health. Ideal for a quick, satisfying lunch or light dinner, it supports sustained energy and muscle maintenance while keeping you full and satisfied.

Ingredients

- 2 to 3 slices of brown bread
- ½ tsp ghee
- Grated carrot - 1 cup
- Onion Chopped - 1 cup
- Capsicum Chopped - 1 cup
- 1 tbsp oil of your choice
- Turmeric - ½ tsp
- Cumin - 1 tsp
- Salt - to taste
- Chili/ Pepper powder - 1 tsp (if required)

Instructions

1. Heat a small pan over medium heat. Add one tablespoon of oil of your choice and fry the grated carrots, chopped onion, and capsicum.
2. While frying, add salt, chili powder, cumin seeds, and turmeric and fry until the vegetables are cooked.

3. Now toast the bread with ½ tsp ghee, place the above-cooked vegetables on the bread, make a sandwich, and enjoy a low-carb and high-fiber sandwich.

2. Moongdal (Green Gram Beans) Pancake

Moongdal pancakes are a high-protein, fiber-rich breakfast option that aids in digestion and keeps you full longer. Made from ground mung beans and spices, these savory pancakes are packed with essential nutrients and are perfect for supporting muscle maintenance and overall energy levels.

Ingredients

- Moong dal - 1 cup
- Ginger, chopped - 1 tbsp
- Turmeric - ½ tsp
- Water ½ cup
- Onion, chopped - 3 tbsp
- Green chili, chopped (if required) - 2 nos
- Cumin - 1 tsp
- Carrot, finely grated - ⅓ cup
- Coriander leaves, chopped - a handful
- Capsicum - ⅓ cup
- Salt - to taste
- Baking Soda - 1 tsp
- Oil - as required

Instructions

1. Let moong dal soak for four to six hours or overnight.
2. Put the drained and soaked moong dal in a blender with water, ginger, and turmeric powder. Process until smooth batter is achieved, adding a little water as needed. The consistency of the batter should be similar to that of the pancake batter.
3. Move the moong dal batter into a mixing basin and add chopped coriander leaves, chopped onions, chopped green chilies, grated

carrots, diced capsicum, and cumin seeds. Stir everything thoroughly. Add the baking soda now and stir slowly.

4. Turn up the heat to medium in a small pan. Spread a few drops of oil evenly after adding them.

5. Transfer a ladleful of the moong dal mixture to the pan, then gently spread it out to create a pancake-like round shape. You can change the thickness to suit your tastes.

6. Drizzle the pancake with a few drops of oil around the edges, cover with a lid, and cook over medium to low heat until the bottom is crispy and golden brown.

7. Turn the pancake over gently to cook the other side.

8. Take the pancake out of the pan and eat the whole meal once it has crisped on both sides.

3. High Protein Tiramisu

High protein tiramisu is a delicious and nutritious twist on the classic dessert, made with protein-rich ingredients like Greek yogurt. This indulgent treat supports muscle maintenance and satisfies your sweet tooth while giving you a healthy dose of protein to keep you full and energized.

Ingredients

- 1 tbsp coffee powder
- 1 tbsp brown sugar
- ½ tsp vanilla essence
- 3 slices of brown bread cut out the edges
- ¼ cup yogurt - unsweetened
- ¼ cup low-fat cottage cheese
- ½ tbsp brown sugar
- ¼ tsp cocoa powder

Instructions

1. Add coffee powder, brown sugar, vanilla essence, and warm water, mix it well and keep it aside.

2. Cut out the brown bread into circles and keep it aside
3. Take a mixer and put yogurt, low-fat cottage cheese, and brown sugar and grind it to a cream texture
4. Take a fresh glass jar, dip the brown bread into the coffee powder mixture, and place it on the jar; add a layer of the yogurt mixture on top of it and do the same for the remaining two slices of the bread, now sprinkle cocoa powder on top of the last layer of yogurt mixture and freeze it for 30 Minutes and enjoy your High protein Tiramisu.

Integrating Healthy Habits Into Your Daily Routine

Maintaining a healthy lifestyle doesn't have to be hard; in fact, it needn't be as hard as it might seem. Making a few modifications to your daily routine will help you start leading a healthier lifestyle.

Here are five healthy habits that you should add to your daily routine:

1. Spending at Least 2 Hours a Week in Strength Training

Strength training is vital to maintain muscle mass and bone density as you age. Dedicate at least two hours weekly to activities like weight lifting, resistance band exercises, or bodyweight workouts. You can break this into shorter sessions, such as 30 minutes four times a week. Find a routine you enjoy and Stick to it, making it a non-negotiable part of your schedule.

2. Walking 10,000 Steps

Start with 5k steps a day. Walking 10 minutes would give you 1000 steps, so walking for 10 minutes after every meal will already give you 3000 steps, and finding another 20 minutes through the day would not be difficult, I hope. Then increase 500 steps every week, and by the time you reach 10k steps, you will start loving these "walks," which will give you your "me time," and it will become a cakewalk in no time.

3. Portion Control, Eating Whole Meals and Avoiding Unhealthy Foods

Eating balanced, whole meals and practicing portion control can significantly impact your health. Focus on including a variety of macronutrients (proteins, fats, carbohydrates) and micronutrients (vitamins, minerals) in your meals. Use smaller plates to help control portions, and ensure each meal includes fiber-rich vegetables, lean proteins, and healthy fats. This approach helps manage weight, supports digestion, and provides sustained energy. Additionally, avoid junk food, oily foods, and limit sugar intake in all forms to reduce the risk of chronic diseases and maintain optimal health.

4. Sleeping Well

Getting enough sleep is critical for general wellness, including mental clarity, mood, and physical recovery. Aim for 7-9 hours of sleep per night. Create a relaxing nighttime routine like reading a book or doing relaxation exercises to let your body know when it's time to wind down. Keep your sleep environment comfortable and free from distractions to promote restful sleep.

5. Drinking Enough Water

Staying hydrated is essential for preserving energy levels, supporting digestion, and keeping your skin healthy. Take a water bottle with you throughout the day to remind yourself to drink regularly. Aim for at least eight glasses of water per day but adjust based on your activity level and climate. Drinking water before eating can also aid in portion control and prevent overeating.

6. Managing stress levels

Managing stress is crucial for maintaining mental and physical health. Practice stress-reducing activities like yoga, meditation, deep breathing exercises, or even hobbies that you enjoy. Ensure you take time for yourself each day to unwind and relax. Keeping stress levels in check can improve your mood, enhance your immune function, and promote overall well-being.

Interactive Reflection Section

1. What changes can you make to your current diet to increase your intake of essential nutrients, particularly fiber and protein?

Consider the foods you currently eat and consider how to incorporate more fiber-rich fruits, vegetables, whole grains, and protein sources like lean meats, beans, and nuts.

Potential changes to increase fiber intake:

_____

_____

Potential changes to increase protein intake:

_____

_____

2. Reflect on one healthy habit you've successfully integrated into your daily routine. How has this habit impacted your lifestyle and wellness?

Think about a healthy habit you've adopted, such as regular exercise, portion control, or staying hydrated. Reflect on how this habit has improved your physical and mental health.

Healthy habit integrated:

_____

_____

Impact on lifestyle and wellness:

_____

_____

FIBER AND PROTEIN INTAKE JOURNAL

Use this space to track your fiber and protein intake, noting any changes in your energy levels, digestion, and overall well-being.

Fiber-Rich Foods Consumed:

Breakfast:

_____

Lunch:

_____

Dinner:

_____

Snacks:

_____

Protein Sources Consumed:

Breakfast:

_____

Lunch:

_____

Dinner:

_____

Snacks:

_____

Notes on Energy Levels, Digestion, and Overall Well-Being:

Energy levels today:

_____

Digestion:

_____

Overall feeling:

_____

Tracking your nutrient intake and new habits can provide valuable insights into your health journey. By reflecting on these changes and monitoring your progress, you can make informed adjustments and continue to improve your overall well-being. Keep using these tools to stay motivated and empowered on your path to a healthier lifestyle.

After learning that balanced whole meals and healthy lifestyle changes will transform you physically and mentally, In the next chapter, we learn the anatomy of an effective workout routine designed for women over 50.

CHAPTER FOUR
Parts Of The Workout/Exercises

Exercising improves bodies, including those of women above 50 and older. The benefits of a fitness routine for seniors include an increase in muscle mass, metabolism, balance, flexibility, endurance, and cardiac capacity, depending on the components of the workout.

With so many exercises available, there is bound to be one that suits the skills or fitness level of any individual. For healthy older adults, a well-rounded fitness routine should incorporate cardio, flexibility, and strength training.

Strength training and flexibility exercises focus on the main muscle groups in the body. For the upper body muscles, these are the shoulders, arms (biceps and triceps), back, Chest, and abdomen. The lower body and legs (glutes, hamstrings, quadriceps, calves) are the main areas of attention.

Seniors with medical issues can also exercise. Ideally, they should first obtain their doctor's approval, with any suggested limitations. When starting a fitness program, people who don't have easy access to medical care should remember to go slowly and carefully.

This chapter is designed to guide you through the essential components of an effective workout and highlight the key equipment that can enhance your exercise routine. As women over 50, understanding how to structure your workouts and investing in the right tools can make all the difference in achieving your fitness goals.

We'll discuss the importance of warming up to prepare your body, the main workout to build strength and endurance, and the cool-down to aid recovery. You'll also discover must-have equipment that can boost your progress and make your workouts more enjoyable. Embrace this knowledge and gear up for a more informed and empowered approach to your fitness regimen.

Warm-Up

Being physically active is crucial no matter what age we are, but how we prepare for physical activity matters more and more as we age. Seniors who exercise regularly can significantly maintain their strength, health, and injury-free lifestyles.

Warm-ups raise body temperature in the core and get the heart, muscles, and joints ready for the demands of exercise. This is especially important in the cooler temperatures when there is a higher chance of heart strain.

What is a Warm-up?

In other words, a warm-up helps your heart, muscles, and joints get ready for exercise by raising your body's core temperature.

You can prevent exercise-related injuries and greatly increase your flexibility by warming up your upper body, lower body, or both. Most significantly, the arteries may be less able to transfer blood at temperatures below 59°, which could impose an excessive amount of strain on the heart.

Ideally, a brief warm-up gives your body the ready-made setup it needs for safe exercise.

Let's look at the ins and outs of a warm-up and why it's so important to your fitness routine.

The Benefits of Warming Up

Walking up a slope causes an increase in your body's core temperature, as shown by the heat you feel. This indicates that your heart is pumping blood into your muscles.

Ignoring the warm-up increases the chance of injury. The muscles and connective tissue, including the muscles in your heart, are not prepared for movement without a warm-up exercise, especially if you are new to exercising.

You can keep yourself safe by beginning your day—or your workout—with a powerful movement that resembles the exercises you are about to perform.

Is Stretching and Warming Up the Same Thing?

Yes and no. Stretching exercises are typically thought of as a "stretch-and-hold" (or static stretching) technique. Although static stretching is a great post-workout movement, the main objective of a warm-up is to move in a manner similar to the activity you are going to perform.

They are referred to as dynamic warm-ups or stretches. Dynamic stretches are similar to the exercise you're preparing for, but they're less strenuous and usually have a limited range of motion.

Since most physical activities include using all or most of the body, it's best to do warm-ups that involve moving your entire body, including your spine, to make sure that all body parts are ready.

Dynamic warm-up exercises that are carefully designed also provide safe and easy challenges to your balance, which improve overall health and fall prevention.

Warm-up exercises offer a quick and efficient approach to incorporating injury prevention into your workout regimen by getting your heart rate up to increase blood flow, prime your muscles for action, and turn on your body's balancing system.

Dynamic Stretching: Stretching during warm up is known as dynamic stretching. This stretching involves moving parts of your body through a full range of motion. This type of stretching is often used as part of a warm-up. Examples include arm circles, leg swings, and torso Twists.

Main Workout: Building Strength

When it comes to functional ability and building strength, several key factors play an essential role in the effectiveness of your main workout. Understanding these elements can help you see how the workouts in chapters 5 and 6 will help you meet your fitness goals, as all the exercises provided are suitable for women over 50.

What are Reps, Sets, Rest Periods, Tempo, and Progressive Overload?

Reps: A rep (repetition) is the number of times you perform a specific exercise movement. For example, lifting a dumbbell from your side to your shoulder and back down once is one rep.

Sets: A set is a group of consecutive reps performed without resting. For instance, if you do ten reps of an exercise, take a short break, and then do ten more reps, you've completed two sets of 10 reps each.

Rest Periods: Rest periods are the breaks you take between sets or exercises. These periods allow your muscles to recover slightly before you continue, which is crucial for maintaining proper form and intensity.

Tempo: Tempo is the speed at which you perform each rep. It includes the time spent on the lifting (concentric) phase, the lowering (eccentric) phase, and any pauses in between. A controlled tempo ensures you perform each movement correctly, minimizing the risk of injury and improving muscle engagement.

Progressive Overload: This is the steady increase of stress placed on your muscles during training. This can be attained by increasing the number of sets or reps, lifting heavier weights, or enhancing the intensity of the exercises. For example, if you did ten reps of an exercise with a specific weight last week, doing 11 reps with the same weight this week is a form of progressive overload.

Importance of Sets, Reps, Rest Periods, Tempo, and Progressive Overload in Building Strength

Sets and Reps: The combination of sets and reps determines the total volume of your workout. For building strength, a common approach is to perform multiple sets with a moderate to low number of reps (e.g., 3-5 sets of 8-12 reps). This helps you focus on lifting heavier weights while maintaining good form, essential for muscle growth and strength.

Rest Periods: Rest periods between sets must be long enough to allow partial recovery but short enough to keep your muscles challenged. Typically, rest periods of 15-20 seconds to 1-2 minutes are recommended for strength training, depending on the time you have for doing the workout. This balance helps you maintain intensity while allowing your muscles to recover and prepare for the next set.

Tempo: Maintaining a consistent and controlled tempo ensures you are effectively engaging the targeted muscles and reducing the risk of injury. For example, a tempo of 2 seconds lifting, 1-second pause, and 2 seconds lowering (2-1-2) can enhance muscle activation and endurance.

Progressive Overload: Adding progressive overload into your training ensures continuous improvement and prevents plateaus. By slowly increasing the demands on your muscles, you force them to adapt and grow stronger. This could be as simple as adding an extra rep or slightly improving the weight you lift each week.

By understanding and putting these ideas into practice, you can create an effective and efficient main workout routine that builds strength and enhances functional ability. Remember, quality over quantity is key— focus on performing each exercise with proper form and control to reduce the possibility of injury and optimize your results.

Compound And Rotational Exercises

As you progress in your fitness journey, it's important to understand the value of compound and Rotational exercises. These movements make your workout more efficient and offer numerous benefits, especially for women over 50.

Compound Exercises: Compound exercises involve multiple muscle joints and groups working together. Examples include squats, deadlifts, and push-ups. These exercises mimic everyday movements, making them incredibly functional and practical. For instance, a squat can help improve your ability to sit and stand, while a deadlift can enhance your ability to safely lift objects from the ground.

Rotational Exercises: Rotational exercises incorporate twisting or turning movements, engaging the core, and improving stability and balance. Examples include Russian Twists, woodchoppers, and medicine ball throws. These exercises are particularly beneficial for maintaining a strong core, which is essential for overall balance and preventing falls.

Including compound and Rotational exercises in your routine increases the effectiveness and efficiency of your workout program. Here's how:

1. Enhanced Muscle Engagement: Compound exercises activate multiple muscle groups simultaneously, which implies you get more out of each movement. This leads to greater muscle activation and strength gains in less time compared to isolation exercises that focus only on one muscle group at a time.

2. Improved Functional Strength: Both compound and Rotational exercises mimic real-life movements, making everyday activities easier and safer. This functional strength is crucial for maintaining independence and minimizing the risk of injuries in daily life.

3. Better Core Stability: Rotational exercises are excellent for building stability and core strength, which are important for balance and posture. A strong core reduces back pain, supports your spine, and enhances overall stability, making all physical activities easier and safer.

4. Efficient Workouts: By engaging multiple muscle groups, these exercises allow you to perform a full-body workout in a shorter time. This efficiency is perfect for busy schedules and ensures you get a comprehensive workout without spending hours in the gym.

5. Enhanced Caloric Burn: Because compound exercises involve more muscle groups, they tend to burn more calories than isolation exercises.

This can be useful for weight management and overall cardiovascular health.

6. Improved Mobility and Flexibility: Rotational movements help enhance muscle flexibility and joint range of motion. This increased mobility is particularly important as you age, helping you maintain an active and agile lifestyle.

By incorporating compound and Rotational exercises into your workout routine, you enhance the overall efficiency and effectiveness of your program. This book includes these exercises to maximize your results.

These movements provide a comprehensive approach to strength training, functional ability, and overall fitness, ensuring you get the most out of your efforts. Embrace these exercises to build strength and improve your daily life, keeping you active, strong, and independent.

Cardiovascular Exercises

Living a healthy lifestyle benefits the mind as much as the body. Aerobic or cardiovascular activity is also a keystone of a healthy lifestyle.

Heart health is more important for seniors than anyone since it protects them against heart disease and prolongs their mobility. That means scheduling a regular cardio workout into your weekly schedule is essential.

Benefits of Cardio Exercises

Adding aerobic activities to your regular fitness routine has numerous advantages, from enhancing heart health to reducing stress and anxiety.

Improves Heart Health: Raising your heart rate makes your heart stronger and more exercised, which can lower the number of beats per minute required to maintain your body getting oxygen.

Aids in Weight Loss: Consistent exercise contributes to gradual calorie burning, which reduces weight and body fat.

Reduces Stress: Physical activity encourages the body to release endorphins, a feel-good hormone that improves mood and lowers stress.

Enhances Memory: Research has shown that regular exercise over time can improve memory and brain function. Increased heart rate and blood flow also supply the brain with nutrients.

Improves Sleep: As we age, most people report difficulty falling asleep. Maintaining an active lifestyle increases both the quantity and quality of sleep.

Older people can try biking, walking, jazz, water aerobics, and other activities for low-impact cardio exercises. When starting again after a layoff or for the first time, if you are new to cardio, you may begin slowly by only completing a few minutes each day. This increases stamina. Add more minutes each week until you reach thirty minutes or more.

Some trainers advise seniors to engage in low-impact aerobic exercise for roughly 150 minutes weekly. To reach this level, some people may decide to work out for 10 or 15 minutes twice or three times a day. You can perform cardio five days a week and take two days off to relax.

Core Strengthening

The core muscles are situated at the center of your body. They extend from your rib cage and go down your pelvis and hips. They extend down to your buttocks and comprise the muscles that support your spine.

These muscles support many important actions and movements, including standing, getting up from a Chair, bending, lifting, and maintaining balance.

Maintaining the right shape of these muscles is essential because of the significance of the movements they support. As you age, your body tends to lose muscular mass and strength.

As a woman above 50, you need to maintain your core strength even more because it's important to maintain proper posture, avoid injuries, and ensure your muscles can support daily tasks for as long as possible.

One of the most important things to keep your core strong is to exercise regularly. Your core is needed for many everyday activities, such as walking and climbing stairs. Your limbs' movements are supported and improved by your core muscles.

Benefits of Core Strengthening Exercises for Seniors

According to research, regular exercise provides numerous other advantages in addition to slowing down the aging process.

Pain control. Older people often experience pain, including lower back pain. Core exercises help control pain and strengthen the muscles in this important area. They occasionally also aid in its reduction.

Enhanced stability and balance. Your general balance and strength are improved, and your spine is supported in large part by your core muscles. This gives you the confidence to perform a variety of actions.

Preventing injury. It takes longer for the body to recover from an injury after a particular age since the body's natural healing process slows down after that point. For this reason, avoiding injuries becomes essential. Regular exercise preserves vital body movements and guards against accidents from falls or other everyday activities.

Increased physical power. According to research, regular exercise can improve an older adult's body strength by up to 30% and help them move a wider range of motion.

Ace your daily chores. You can go about your regular activities with conviction when your body is in good shape. A well-developed core enhances your ability to react quickly and boosts your self-confidence when performing various tasks like walking down a hill or climbing stairs, among other daily activities.

Cool Down/Stretching

Cooling down and stretching are vital parts of any workout routine, particularly for women over 50. These practices help your body transition from the high intensity of your workout to a state of rest, aiding in recovery and preventing injuries.

Cool Down: The cool-down phase typically involves gradually reducing the intensity of your exercise, allowing your heart rate and breathing to return to normal. This helps prevent dizziness and promotes a steady recovery of pre-exercise heart rate and blood Pressure.

Stretching: Stretching focuses on increasing flexibility and maintaining the range of motion in your joints. This is especially important as we age to keep our muscles pliable and reduce the risk of stiffness and injury.

Static Stretching: Stretching during cool down is known as static stretching. This stretching involves holding a stretch for a set period, usually between 15-60 seconds. This helps lengthen muscles and improve flexibility. Examples include hamstring stretches, calf stretches, and shoulder stretches.

Benefits of Stretching

Improved Flexibility: Regular stretching helps lengthen muscles and tendons, increasing flexibility and range of motion.

Improved Circulation: Stretching improves blood flow to the muscles, which can reduce soreness and help with muscle recovery.

Stress Relief: Stretching can help relieve tension and stress, promoting relaxation and overall well-being.

Tips for Safe Stretching

Warm Up First: Always warm up your muscles with light aerobic activity before stretching to prevent injuries. This can be as simple as a few minutes of walking or gentle Jogging.

Proper Technique: Focus on proper form to ensure you target the right muscles and prevent injury. Avoid bouncing or jerking movements during stretching; stretch in a smooth, controlled manner.

Listen to Your Body: Stretch to the point of mild discomfort, not pain. Overstretching can cause muscle strain or injuries. Pay attention to your body's signals and avoid pushing too hard.

Incorporating regular stretching and a cool-down phase into your workout program can significantly improve your flexibility, minimize muscle soreness, and prevent injuries. Remember, listening to your body and focusing on appropriate form and technique is key to reaping the full benefits of these practices.

Safety Tips And Injury Prevention

National Institute on Aging reported that older adults should engage in moderate-intensity workouts for at least 2.5 hours (150 minutes) every week. It is not necessary—in fact, it is not advised—to complete it all in a single day.

Alternatively, break up your activity-based exercise into at least three days, and dedicate at least two of those days to strengthening your muscles with sit-ups, weightlifting, or any other acceptable and safe exercise.

Tips to stay safe and make the most of your workouts:

- Start with easier workouts and work your way up to more challenging ones as your strength and endurance improve. Stretching and lower-intensity exercises are particularly beneficial for increasing flexibility.
- Always warm up before beginning to increase blood flow and reduce the risk of injury. Whether you're working out inside or outside, make sure the environment around you is clear of debris and obstructions that could trip you up.
- Put on shoes and clothes appropriate for the activity you are doing. If you intend to work out outside, pick a time of day when it's warmer in the winter or cooler in the summer. If the weather seems bad, move your workouts indoors.
- There are a lot of exercises you can perform while lying or sitting down if you have trouble with your balance or limited mobility. In addition to providing a whole-body workout, these exercises help you develop physical strength and can also help you focus and de-stress.
- Another form of exercise that is especially good for elderly citizens is aqua therapy. Because the water keeps you buoyant, you can get a tremendous aerobic workout without straining your joints.

58

- Drink plenty of water before, during, and after your workout. You should drink more water to replace the fluids your body loses while you exercise, even if you don't feel thirsty. Hydration is especially important for seniors.

Equipment To Buy For Home Workouts

Creating a home workout setup can be an excellent investment in your health and fitness, providing convenience and flexibility. Here are some essential pieces of equipment to help you build an effective and versatile home gym specifically tailored for women over 50.

1. A Good Thick Mat

A high-quality, thick mat is a must-have for any home workout setup. It provides a comfortable, non-slip surface for exercises, protects your joints during floor work, and offers cushioning for your back and Knees. Look for mats at least 1/4 inch thick for adequate support and comfort.

2. Pairs of Dumbbells (2LBS to 10LBS or 1KG to 5KG)

Dumbbells are incredibly versatile and essential for strength training. Investing in pairs of dumbbells ranging from 2LBS to 10LBS (1KG to 5KG) allows you to perform various exercises targeting different muscle groups. Start with little weights and gradually increase as you build confidence and strength.

3. 4KG Kettlebell

A 4KG kettlebell is perfect for adding dynamic movements to your routine, such as kettlebell swings, goblet squats, and Turkish get-ups. These exercises use multiple muscle groups and improve functional strength, stability, and cardiovascular endurance.

4. Bamboo Stick or PVC Pipe

A bamboo Stick or PVC pipe is helpful for mobility exercises and improving flexibility. It can be used for shoulder dislocations, stretching, and balance exercises, helping to maintain joint health and range of motion.

5. Pilates Band

Pilates bands are excellent for low-impact resistance training, adding an extra challenge to your Pilates or stretching routines. They are lightweight and portable and can be used to target various muscle groups, enhancing strength and flexibility.

6. Resistance Band

Resistance bands are another versatile piece of equipment. They provide adjustable resistance for strength training exercises. They come in different resistance levels, making them suitable for all fitness levels. Use them for exercises like bicep Curls, leg Presses, and Chest Presses to add variety to your workouts.

7. Mini Loop Bands

Mini loop bands are small, circular bands that can be used for a range of lower and upper body exercises, such as squats, leg lifts, glute Bridges and Triceps extensions. They are particularly effective for targeting the hips, glutes, thighs, upper back and arms, helping to build strength and stability in these areas.

8. Pair of 2LBS or 1KG Ankle Weights

Ankle weights can add a challenge to your lower body workouts, improving muscle strength and endurance. They are ideal for exercises like leg lifts, donkey kicks, and walking, helping to increase the intensity of your exercises and promote muscle growth.

Investing in these pieces of equipment can create a comprehensive and flexible home workout setup that meets your fitness needs. Each item serves a unique purpose, allowing you to perform several exercises that build strength, improve flexibility, and enhance overall fitness.

With this setup, you can enjoy the ease of working out at home while achieving your health and wellness goals. Remember to start with lighter weights and gently increase the intensity as you progress, always focusing on appropriate form and technique to prevent injuries.

Interactive Section: Reflect And Plan

Reflecting on your current fitness habits and planning for future improvements is key to staying motivated and progressing in your fitness journey. Take some time to answer these questions and think about enhancing your home workout setup and routine.

Questions to Reflect On

1. What equipment have you used earlier, and what other equipment do you consider investing in?

_____

_____

_____

2. Have you tried mobility exercises earlier? If yes, which ones?

_____

_____

_____

3. What cardiovascular exercises do you enjoy the most?

_____

_____

_____

4. Have you tried stretching earlier? How has it benefited you?

_____

_____

_____

JOURNAL YOUR THOUGHTS AND EXERCISES

Use this space to jot down your thoughts and ideas about the exercises and equipment mentioned in this chapter. Reflect on the exercises you already know, those you enjoy, and any new ones you're excited to try. This can help you create a personalized and efficient workout routine that fits your needs and preferences.

Exercises I Know and Enjoy:

_____

_____

_____

_____

Exercises I Want to Try:

_____

_____

_____

_____

Thoughts and Reflections:

_____

_____

_____

_____

By taking the time to reflect and plan, you can make better decisions about your fitness journey and ensure that you invest in equipment and exercises to help you achieve your goals. Embrace this process to stay committed and motivated to your health and well-being.

The next chapter is the actual exciting chapter that you are waiting to read and implement. This is where 12 months' ready-made workout plans plus 6 HIIT programs are included with links to YouTube videos. These 12 months' readymade workout plans and the 6 HIIT programs include all the parts of a workout as mentioned in Chapter 4, and each workout plan can be completed in just 30 minutes and can be performed in the comfort of your home or anywhere else, all you need is a mat, a pair of dumbbells or a resistance band.

CHAPTER FIVE
Ready-Made Workout Programs At Home

A re you ready to take control of your fitness journey easily and efficiently? This is the chapter you've been waiting for—the one that will kickstart your path to a healthier, stronger you! We'll guide you through the different parts of a workout, from warm-up to cool-down, and introduce you to the essential equipment for a home gym. Plus, you'll find 12 ready-made workout programs—one for each month of the year— that fit seamlessly into your lifestyle, requiring just 30 minutes a day, four days a week. These plans are crafted to help you build strength, improve flexibility, and boost overall health, all from the comfort of your home. Get ready to embrace your fitness journey and transform your life!

Essential Pre-Workout Instructions

Before you begin your fitness journey, it's crucial to prioritize safety and ensure you're prepared. Follow these steps to get the most out of your workouts:

1. **Safety First:** You know your body best, so progress or regress based on your fitness levels.
2. **Workout Videos with QR Codes:** You can access all of the workout videos by scanning the given QR codes.
3. **Pre-Workout Preparation:** Watch the YouTube videos for guidance first, then follow along with the prescribed sets and reps.

For the best experience, view the videos on a laptop or switch to landscape mode if using a mobile.

4. **Listening to Your Body:** On days when you feel tired or strained, opt for a lighter workout. You can always choose Month 1, Week 1 exercises to warm up and keep moving.

5. **General Instructions/Technique/Form:** Watch the YouTube video for general instructions before starting any workout. The QR code to this video is provided below.

6. **Core Engagement:** Before starting any workout, pull your navel toward your spine to fully engage your core muscles. Imagine someone has tied a rope to your belly button and they are pulling it towards your spine to ensure you are engaging your core/abdominal muscles fully.

7. **Pelvic Alignment:** Give an anterior tilt to your pelvic girdle to ensure your spine is straight and there's no lower back arching.

8. **Shoulder Position:** Keep your shoulders retracted and depressed. Roll back your shoulders and keep your shoulder blades together. Imagine you are pushing your shoulder blades inside the back pockets of your jeans; this will ensure you are not hunching and are engaging your Lat muscles (side upper back muscles), which will protect your spine when you lift heavy and in the exercises that you have to bend forward.

9. **Breathing:** Always breathe in through your nose and out through your mouth. Breathe out against gravity, such as exhaling when rising from a squat.

10. **Focus:** While working out, focus on the mind-muscle connection and leave everything else behind – forget about cooking dinner, solving office problems, or even what to watch on Netflix next

Specific Exercise Form And Technique

We've provided detailed instructions for a few key exercises that might be challenging to master just by watching a video. These exercises are crucial for building strength, improving form, and ensuring you get the most out of your workouts. While most of the exercises can be easily followed along with our YouTube videos, these specific ones require a bit more attention to technique and detail. Dive in, carefully read these instructions, and feel confident as you tackle these important movements. Remember, mastering these will set a solid foundation for your fitness journey!

Lying on Your Back Exercises: For dead bugs, glute Bridges, and other core exercises:

- To engage your core, bring your navel towards your spine.
- Tilt your pelvic girdle to ensure your back is flat on the mat.
- Maintain steady breathing throughout.

Quadruped (4-Legged Position) Exercises:

- Ensure hands are directly under your shoulders and Knees under your hips.
- Keep your navel pulled to your spine.

IYWTOs:

- Form the alphabets I, Y, W, T, and O with your arms to strengthen your scapula (shoulder blades).

Squats:

- Stand up with your legs Hip width apart, feet parallel to each other
- Naval pulled to spine
- Hinge your hip and go down as though you are sitting on a Chair, activating your quadriceps (front of your thighs)

- Ensure your Chest is up and not leaning too forward - imagine a big smiley on your t-shirt; when you squat, that smiley should be entirely visible.
- To begin with, go down as much as possible only; with practice, you can squat deeper.
- Then, come up by activating your glutes

Sumo Squats:

- The only difference between Squats and Sumo Squats is that Sumos have wider than hip-width stance with your legs and the toes are pointing outside
- Ensure your Knees are in line with your toes and not caving in.

Deadlift

- Stand up with your legs Hip width apart, feet parallel to each other
- Hold the dumbbells in each hand with palms facing your thighs
- Naval pulled to spine to engage your core, pelvic tilted to keep a neutral spine
- Now hinge your hip slowly, bend your Knees and lean forward (still keeping your core engaged and spine neutral; do not hunch) and go down to Touch your toes
- Push through your heels and maintain a straight hip range to return to the starting position. The dumbbells will move back up along your legs.
- At the top of the movement, squeeze your glutes (butt muscles) to ensure full extension of your hips.

DB Hip Thrusts

- Sit on the ground with your back against the bench/Chair
- Place a dumbbell across your hips.

- Rest your upper back (just below your shoulder blades) on the bench/Chair
- Place your feet flat on the ground, shoulder-width apart, with your Knees bent.
- Naval Pulled to spine, push through your heels to lift your hips toward the ceiling.
- Lift your hips until your shoulders to Knees are in a straight line. At the peak of the exercise, your Knees should be 90 degrees bent.
- At the top, squeeze your glutes (butt muscles) hard and hold for a moment.
- Slowly lower your hips back down to the ground, but do not let them Touch the ground completely. Keep the tension in your glutes.

Step up

- Stand upright, facing the Chair with your legs hip-width apart
- Naval pulled to spine and neutral spine
- Hold the dumbbells in each hand with palms facing your thighs
- Place your right foot on the Chair with your full feet and your heel supported
- Push through your right foot and DO NOT push through your legs that are down, fully engaging your quads and glutes on the right leg
- Lift your left foot to meet the other foot on the Chair, standing tall.
- Step down your left foot and repeat this for said no. of repetitions on the right, followed by the left foot.

Romanian Deadlift (RDL)

- Stand up with your legs Hip width apart, feet parallel to each other
- Hold the dumbbells in each hand with palms facing your thighs

- Naval pulled to the spine to engage your core, pelvic tilted to keep a neutral spine
- Knees are soft; do not lock your Knees
- Now hinge your hip slowly, imagine a wall behind you, now try Touching your butt to the wall, push your hip back as much as possible, and slide the dumbbells on your legs until you reach just below your Knees (still keeping your core engaged and spine neutral, do not hunch) feeling a good stretch in your hamstrings (back of your thighs)
- Avoid rounding your shoulders. Keep them back and down
- Push through your heels and maintain straight hips to return to the starting position, loading the hamstrings. The dumbbells will move back up along your legs.

Straight Leg Deadlift (SDL)

- Stand up with your legs Hip width apart, feet parallel to each other
- Hold the dumbbells in each hand with palms facing your thighs
- Naval pulled to spine to engage your core, pelvic tilted to keep a neutral spine
- Knees are soft; do not lock your Knees
- Push back your hips as you lower the dumbbells towards the ground. Your torso will naturally lean forward.
- Lower the dumbbells to your ankles until you feel a stretch in your hamstrings.
- Avoid rounding your shoulders. Keep them back and down
- Push through your heels and maintain straight hips to return to the starting position. The dumbbells will move back up along your legs.

Reverse lunge.

- Take a big step backward with your right foot.

- Bend both Knees to lower your body. Your right Knee should be just above the floor, and your left Knee should be at a 90-degree angle directly above your ankle.
- Maintain an upright torso and evenly distribute your weight.
- Push through your left heel to return to the starting position, bringing your right foot forward.
- In the video, I have shown one leg going back into a lunge. However, the work is happening on the glutes/quads of the leg that is stationary.

Breathing Tips

- Breathing: Always breathe in through your nose and out through your mouth.
- Timing: Breathe out against gravity; for example, exhale when rising from a squat.

By following these guidelines and watching the instructional videos, you'll be well-prepared to start your workouts safely and effectively. Let's get moving and achieve those fitness goals!

Your Ultimate Home Workout Guide

Welcome to your comprehensive fitness journey with 12 ready-made, effective workout plans designed to fit seamlessly into your lifestyle. Spend just 30 minutes a day, four days a week, and transform your body and mind. Here's what you can expect:

Maximize Strength: These plans focus on fat loss and muscle building.

Improve Mobility and Flexibility: Keep your body agile and limber.

Floor-Free Alternatives: Options for those who prefer not to exercise on the floor.

Variety of Equipment: Exercises using different equipment to prevent boredom and promote muscle adaptation.

WORKOUT COMPONENTS

Each workout plan includes:

- Warm-Up: Prepares your body for exercise.
- Main Workout: Targets different muscle groups with compound and Rotational movements.
- Core Strengthening and Stability: Builds a strong, stable core.
- Full Body Conditioning: Comprehensive exercises for overall fitness.
- HIIT and Cardiovascular Movements: Boosts heart health and burns calories.

Every workout program details the exercise group (e.g., warm-up, heart raisers, main workout, stretching), number of reps and sets, and the time required.

There are QR codes linked to YouTube videos for all of the exercise demonstrations. The videos demonstrate the correct form and technique only, so you won't be working out along with them. Instead, watch and learn the proper form, then perform the prescribed reps and sets outlined in the book's workout program. This way, you can ensure you're doing each exercise correctly and safely, maximizing your results!

GETTING STARTED

- Absolute Beginners: Start from Month 1.
- Experienced Intermediate Exercisers: Begin from Month 3 for a structured program.
- Initial Equipment: Start with water bottles for the first two months, but investing in a pair of dumbbells will significantly enhance your workout experience.
- Progressive Overload: Once comfortable with 1kg dumbbells, gradually move to 2kg dumbbells, performing at least 5-6 reps

before switching back to 1kg to complete the set. The same applies to resistance bands.

EQUIPMENT GUIDE FOR EACH MONTH

Month 1: Body weight, Water bottles or Light dumbbells

Month 2: Water bottles or Light dumbbells

Month 3: Water bottles or Light dumbbells

Month 4: Mini Loop Bands

Month 5: Bamboo Stick for mobility, Dumbbells, and Ankle weights

Month 6: Resistance band and Pilates band

Month 7: Dumbbells, Body weight, Ankle Weights, Mini Loop Bands, Bamboo Stick

Month 8: Dumbbells, Body weight, Ankle Weights, Mini Loop Bands, Bamboo Stick, Kettlebell, Pilates Band, Resistance Band

Month 9: Dumbbells, Mini Loop Bands, Resistance Band

Month 10: Dumbbells & Resistance Band Mix (Full Body)

Month 11: Dumbbells and Body Weight

Month 12: Dumbbells and Body Weight (Advanced)

KEY TERMS AND TIPS

- DB: Dumbbell
- BW: Body Weight
- OH: Overhead
- RDL: Romanian Deadlift
- Lat: Latissimus Dorsi (A large, flat muscle on the back that helps in   the movement of the shoulders and arms)

- Rest Period: Take at least 15-20 seconds rest/break between each set

You will see results when you follow a particular program for at least four weeks continuously before moving on to the next one. Changing exercises every day confuses the muscles but shocking them every four weeks helps build them better.

Embrace this journey and enjoy the rewards of a structured, varied, and effective workout program tailored to your needs.

THE WORKOUT PROGRAMS

Month 1, Week 1, Day 1-4

Group	Exercise	No. of Reps	No. of Sets	Time Required to Perform	QR code for Video
Upper Body	Neck Side to Side	6	2	12 Minutes	
	Neck looks down to the Chest and looks straight	6	2		
	Neck goes "U" and look back	6	2		
	Shoulder Rotation Backward and Forward	8	2		
	Hands Up & Down	8	2		
	Hands Crossovers	8	2		
	Small Arm Circles - Clockwise & Anti Clockwise	6 both ways	2		
	BW Shoulder Press		2		
	Shoulder Touches	8	2		
	Overhead Back Touches	8 each hand	2		
	Finger Clenches	10	2		
	Wrist Rotation - Clockwise & Anti Clockwise	8 both ways	2		
	Side Bending with Hands by your Ears	5 each side	2		
	Cross Hands-on Shoulders with Twisting	5 each side	2		
	Hip Rotation	5 each side	2		

Month 1, Week 1, Day 1-4 (Continuation)

Group	Exercise	No. of Reps	No. of Sets	Time Required to Perform	QR code for Video
Lower Body	Standing Toe Touch	8	2	10 Minutes	
	High Knee Marching (with Support)	5 each side	2		
	Butt Kick Marching (With support)	5 each side	2		
	Lateral Single-leg Raises	5 each side	2		
	Front and Back Swings	5 each side	2		
	Squatting on Chair	10	2		
	Heel Raises	15	2		
	Seated Ankle Rotation - Clockwise and Anti Clockwise	6 both ways	2		

Month 1, Week 1, Day 1-4 (Continuation)

Group	Exercise	No. of Reps	No. of Sets	Time Required to Perform	QR code for Video
Heart Raisers	Marching without support - increase speed	30 seconds	2	5 Minutes, including rest periods	
	Slow On-the-spot Jogging	30 seconds	2		
	Step Touch with Hand Movement	30 seconds	2		
Stretching	Seated Chest Stretch	20 seconds	2	5 Minutes	
	Seated Neck Stretch	20 seconds	2		
	Standing Triceps Stretch	20 seconds	2		
	Seated Arm Stretch	20 seconds	2		
	Seated Shoulder Stretch	20 seconds	2		
	Seated Lumbar Stretch	20 seconds	2		
	Seated Thigh Stretch	20 seconds	2		
	Calf Stretch	20 seconds each side	2		
	Breathing	30 seconds	2		

Month 1, Week 2-4, Day 1 – Upper Body (Start with 1 kg dumbbells or water bottle)

Please scan this QR code for the YouTube Video

Group	Exercise	No. of Reps	No. of Sets	Time Required to Perform
Warm-Up	Neck Side to Side	8	2	8 minutes, including rest periods
	Neck looks down to the Chest and looks straight	8	2	
	Neck goes "U" and look back	8	2	
	Shoulder Rotation Backward and Forward	10 each backward & forward	2	
	Hands Crossovers	10	2	
	Small Arm Circles - Clockwise & Anti Clockwise	10	2	
Heart Raisers	Marching without support - increase speed	30 seconds	2	4 minutes, including rest periods
	Slow On-the-spot Jogging	30 seconds	2	
	Step Touch with Hand Movement	30 seconds	2	
Main Workout	Seated IYWTO (body weight)	8	2	14 Minutes
	Seated BW/DB/water bottle Shoulder Press	8	3	
	DB/Water bottle Bicep Curl	8	3	
	DB/Water bottle Halo	8	3	
Stretching	Seated Chest Stretch	20 Seconds	2	4 Minutes
	Seated Shoulder Stretch	20 seconds each side	1	
	Seated Arm Stretch	20 seconds each side	1	

77

Month 1, Week 2-4, Day 2 – Lower Body (Start with 1 kg dumbbells or water bottle)

Please scan this QR code for the YouTube Video

Group	Exercise	No. of Reps	No. of Sets	Time Required to Perform
Warm-Up	Standing Toe Touch	10	1	7 minutes, including rest periods
	Chair Seated Cat Camel	10	2	
	Butt Kick Marching (With support)	10	2	
	Lateral Single-leg Raises	10 Each side	2	
	Seated Ankle Rotation - Clockwise and Anti Clockwise	10 (5 each direction) & both legs	1	
Heart Raisers	Toe Tap Jacks	30 seconds	2	4 minutes, including rest periods
	on-the-spot Jogging	30 seconds	2	
	Step Touch with Hand Movement	30 seconds	2	
Main Workout	Squatting on the Chair	10	3	15 Minutes
	Crossing the Hurdles (2 variations)	at least 4 hurdles, 6 rounds	3	
	Seated Leg Extension (body weight)	10	3	
	Standing Single-leg Curls	10 each leg	3	
Stretching	Seated Thigh Stretch	20 seconds each leg	1	4 Minutes
	Standing Single-leg Knee Hug with wall support	20 seconds each leg	1	
	Standing Calf Stretch	20 seconds each leg	1	

Month 1, Week 2-4, Day 3 – Upper Body (Start with 1 kg dumbbells or water bottle)

Please scan this QR code for the YouTube Video

Group	Exercise	No. of Reps	No. of Sets	Time Required to Perform
Warm-Up	3-way Neck Stretch	8	2	6 Minutes
	Hands Up & Down	10	2	
	Overhead Back Touches	8 each hand	2	
	Wrist Rotation - Clockwise & Anti Clockwise	8 both ways	1	
	Hands by the side of your ears and side bending	8 each side	2	
Heart Raisers	Marching without support - increase speed	30 seconds	2	4 Minutes
	Slow On-the-spot Jogging	30 seconds	2	
	Step Touch with Hand Movement	30 seconds	2	
Main Workout	Seated Lateral Raises (body weight)	10	3	15 Minutes
	DB/water bottle Chest Front Press	10	3	
	DB/water bottle Shrugs	10	3	
	DB/water bottle Triceps Overhead Extension	10	3	
Stretching	Seated Shoulder Stretch	20 Seconds each hand	1	4 Minutes
	Seated Chest Stretch	20 Seconds	1	
	Standing Triceps Stretch	20 seconds each side	1	

Month 1, Week 2-4, Day 4 – Lower Body (Start with 1 kg dumbbells or water bottle)

Please scan this QR code for the YouTube Video

Group	Exercise	No. of Reps	No. of Sets	Time Required to Perform
Warm-Up	Seated Cat Camel	10	2	5 to 6 Minutes
	High Knee Marching (with Support)	10	2	
	Lateral Single-leg Raises	10 Each side	2	
	Seated Ankle Rotation - Clockwise and Anti Clockwise	10 (5 each direction) & both legs	1	
Heart Raisers	Toe Tap Jacks	30 seconds	2	4 Minutes
	on-the-spot Jogging	30 seconds	2	
	Step Touch with Hand Movement	30 seconds	2	
Main Workout	3-way Pendulum Legs with Chair support	10 each side	3	12 to 15 Minutes
	Cross Marching	10 each side	2	
	Seated Leg Raises	8	3	
	Heel Raises	15	3	
Stretching	Seated Thigh Stretch	20 seconds each leg	2	5 Minutes
	Standing single-leg Knee Hug with wall support	20 seconds each leg	1	
	Standing Calf Stretch	20 seconds each leg	2	

Month 2, Week 1-4, Day 1 - Lower Body (Start with 1 kg dumbbells or water bottle)

Please scan this QR code for the YouTube Video

Group	Exercise	No. of Reps	No. of Sets	Time Required to Perform
Warm-Up	Hip Rotation - Clockwise and Anticlockwise	8 each side	2	7 to 8 Minutes
	Lateral Single-leg Raises	8 each side	2	
	Front and Back Swings	8 each side	2	
	Seated Ankle Rotation - Clockwise and Anti Clockwise	8 both ways	2	
Main Workout	Quadruped Cat Camel (on the bed/mat)	10	3	15 Minutes
	DB Squatting on the Chair	10	3	
	Glute Bridges (on the bed/mat)	10	3	
	Deadbug Holds (on the bed/mat)	10 (5 count holds)	2	
Heart Raisers	On-the-spot Jogging	30 seconds work, 15 seconds rest	2	3 Minutes
	On-the-spot high Knee marching (increase the speed)	30 seconds work, 15 seconds rest	2	
Stretching	Standing Knee Hug with wall support	20 seconds hold	1	4 Minutes
	Seated Thigh Stretch	20 seconds hold each side	2	
	Standing Calf Stretch	20 seconds hold each side	2	

Month 2, Week 1-4, Day 2 - Upper Body (Start with 1 kg dumbbells or water bottle)

Please scan this QR code for the YouTube Video

Group	Exercise	No. of Reps	No. of Sets	Time Required to Perform
Warm-Up	3-way Neck Stretch	10	1	5 to 6 Minutes
	Hands Crossovers	10	2	
	Small Arm Circles - Clockwise & Anti Clockwise	10 both ways	2	
	Overhead Back Touches	10 each hand	2	
Main Workout	Lying down DB/water bottle Chest Press (on the bed/mat)	10	3	17 Minutes
	DB/water bottle Lateral raises to front raise	10	3	
	DB/water bottle Triceps Overhead Extension	10	3	
	Lying down Toe Taps (on the bed/mat)	10 total (5 each side)	3	
Heart Raisers	Step Touch with Hand Movement (increase the speed)	30 seconds work, 15 seconds rest	2	3 Minutes
	Slow Skipping	30 seconds work, 15 seconds rest	2	
Stretching	Seated Chest Stretch	20 seconds hold	1	4 Minutes
	Seated Shoulder Stretch	20 seconds hold each side	1	
	Standing Triceps Stretch	20 seconds hold each side	1	

Month 2, Week 1-4, Day 3 - Lower Body (Start with 1 kg dumbbells or water bottle)

Please scan this QR code for the YouTube Video

Group	Exercise	No. of Reps	No. of Sets	Time Required to Perform
Warm-Up	Hip Rotation - Clockwise and Anticlockwise	10 each side	2	5 Minutes
	Standing Toe Touch	10	1	
	Butt Kick Marching (With support)	10 each side	2	
	Seated Ankle Rotation - Clockwise and Anti Clockwise	8 both ways each leg	2	
Main Workout	Clamshells (on the bed/mat)	10 each leg	3	17 Minutes
	DB/water bottle Glute Bridges (on the bed/mat)	10	3	
	Seated BW Single-leg Extension	12	3	
	DB Deadbug Leg Extension	10	3	
Heart Raisers	Toe Tap Jacks (increase the speed)	30 seconds work, 15 seconds rest	2	3 Minutes
	On-the-spot High Knee marching (increase the speed)	30 seconds work, 15 seconds rest	2	
Stretching	Standing Hamstring Stretch	20 seconds hold	1	4 Minutes
	Standing Calf Stretch	20 seconds hold each side	1	
	Standing Quad Stretch (with Support)	20 seconds hold each side	1	

Month 2, Week 1-4, Day 4 - Upper Body (Start with 1 kg dumbbells or water bottle)

Please scan this QR code for the YouTube Video

Group	Exercise	No. of Reps	No. of Sets	Time Required to Perform
Warm-Up	3-way Neck stretch	10 each	1	5 to 6 Minutes
	Hands Up & Down	10	2	
	Shoulder Touches	10	2	
	Hip Hinged Ys & Ts	10 each	2	
Main Workout	DB/water bottle Upright Row	10	3	15 Minutes
	Superman single-side opposite Limb lift (on the bed/mat)	10 total (5 each side)	3	
	DB/water bottle Bicep Curls	10 total (5 each side)	3	
	Heel Slides (on the bed/mat)	10 total (5 each side)	3	
Heart Raisers	Step up (1st step of staircase/low height stool, stepper) Use only 1 leg in 1st set and use the other leg in 2nd set	30 seconds work, 15 seconds rest	2	3 Minutes
	Step Touch with Hand Movement (increase the speed)	30 seconds work, 15 seconds rest	2	
Stretching	Sphinx Pose (on the bed/mat)	20 seconds hold	1	5 Minutes
	Child's Pose (on the bed/mat)	20 seconds hold	2	
	Seated Arm Stretch	20 seconds hold	1	

Month 3, week 1-4, Day 1 – Lower Body (Increase to 2KG Dumbbells)

Please scan this QR code for the YouTube Video

Group	Exercise	No. of Reps	No. of Sets	Time Required to Perform
Warm-Up	Quadruped Cat Camel (on the bed /mat)	8	2	5 Minutes
	Standing Hip Openers (take the support of Chair/wall)	8 each side	2	
	Hip Hinging	8	2	
Main Workout	Air Squats (take support of Chair)	10	3	17 Minutes
	Quadruped single-leg hamstring Curl (on the bed/mat)	10 each leg	3	
	Weighted/DB Glute Bridges	12	3	
	Adductor Ball/Pillow Squeeze	8 (5 count holds)	3	
Heart Raisers	Step Up & Down (on stepper/on stairs 1st step)	30 seconds work, 15 seconds rest	2	3 Minutes
	Butt Kicks (with the support of the Chair) - increase the speed	30 seconds work, 15 seconds rest	2	
Stretching	Lying down Knee Hug	20 seconds, hold each side	2	5 Minutes
	Lying down Hamstring stretch with Resistance Band/thin towel/scarf	20 seconds hold each side	2	
	Wide-legged seated forward bend	20 seconds hold	2	

Month 3, week 1-4, Day 2 – Upper Body (Increase to 2KG Dumbbells)

Please scan this QR code for the YouTube Video

Group	Exercise	No. of Reps	No. of Sets	Time Required to Perform
Warm-Up	Small Arm Circles - Clockwise & Anticlockwise (quick ones)	10 each side	2	5 Minutes
	BW Shoulder Press	10	2	
	Overhead Back Touches	10 each hand	2	
	Hands Crossovers	12	2	
Main Workout	DB Chair seated Shoulder Press	12	3	17 Minutes
	DB Lying down Chest Press (lying down on mat/bed)	10	3	
	DB Chair seated OH Extension	10	3	
	Lying down Toe Taps (on the bed/mat)	12 total (6 each leg)	3	
Heart raisers	Jumping Jack	30 seconds work, 15 seconds rest	2	3 Minutes
	On-the-spot Jogging	30 seconds work, 15 seconds rest	2	
Stretching	Standing Shoulder Stretch	20 seconds hold each side	2	5 Minutes
	Wall-assisted Chest Stretch	20 seconds hold each side	2	
	Standing Triceps Stretch	20 seconds hold each side	2	

Month 3, week 1-4, Day 3 – Lower Body (Increase to 2KG Dumbbells)

Please scan this QR code for the YouTube Video

Group	Exercise	No. of Reps	No. of Sets	Time Required to Perform
Warm-Up	Mountain Pose Hamstring Stretch	10 each leg	2	5 Minutes
	Dynamic Quad Stretch (take Chair/wall support)	10 each leg	2	
	Standing Ankle Rotation - Clockwise and Anti Clockwise	10 both ways each leg	1	
Main workout	DB Goblet Squats	10	3	17 Minutes
	Quad Rockers	10	2	
	Heel Raises (3-way foot variation)	10 each variation	3	
	Side Plank (Knee down)	30 seconds each side	3	
Heart raisers	Side-to-side Shuffle	30 seconds work, 15 seconds rest	2	3 Minutes
	Jumping Jacks	30 seconds work, 15 seconds rest	2	
Stretching	Standing Static Quad Stretch	30 seconds each leg	2	5 Minutes
	Standing Calves Stretch	30 seconds each leg	2	

Month 3, week 1-4, Day 4 – Upper Body (Increase to 2KG Dumbbells)

Please scan this QR code for the YouTube Video

Group	Exercise	No. of Reps	No. of Sets	Time Required to Perform
Warm-Up	Quadruped T spine Rotation	8 each side	2	4 Minutes
	Lying down Y's & Ts	10 each	1	
	Shoulder Touches	10	2	
Main workout	Single-arm DB Rowing	10 each side	3	17 Minutes
	Lying down Os	8	3	
	DB Hammer Curl	10	3	
	DB Deadbug holds	10 (5 count holds)	3	
Heart raisers	Foot Fire	30 seconds work, 15 seconds rest	2	3 Minutes
	Step Up & Down (on stepper/on stairs 1st step)	30 seconds work, 15 seconds rest	2	
Stretching	Child's Pose hold	30 seconds hold	1	5 Minutes
	Wall-assisted Lat Stretch	30 seconds hold	1	
	Standing Arm Stretch	20 seconds hold each arm	2	

Month 4, Week 1-4, Day 1 – Upper Body (Mini Band/Loop Band Workout)

Please scan this QR code for the YouTube Video

Group	Exercise	No. of Reps	No. of Sets	Time Required to Perform
Warm-Up	Hinging/Seated Ys and Ts	10 each	2	7 Minutes
	Quadruped T Spine Rotation	10 each side	2	
	BW Shoulder Press	10	2	
Main workout	Banded Single-arm shoulder Press	10 each side	3	17 Minutes
	Banded Seated Single-arm lateral raise	10 each side	3	
	Banded Seated Single-arm Rowing	10 each side	3	
	Banded Single-arm Lat pulldown	10 each side	3	
	Flutter kicks	30 seconds	2	
Heart Raisers	Zumba Dance Move	30 seconds work, 15 seconds rest	2	3 Minutes
	Butt Kicks	30 seconds work, 15 seconds rest	2	
Stretching	Puppy dog Pose	20 seconds hold	1	3 Minutes
	Wall-assisted Lat Stretch	20 seconds hold	1	
	Standing Shoulder Stretch	20 seconds hold each side	1	

Month 4, Week 1-4, Day 2 – Lower Body (Mini Band/Loop Band Workout)

Please scan this QR code for the YouTube Video

Group	Exercise	No. of Reps	No. of Sets	Time Required to Perform
Warm-Up	Seated Leg Raises	10 reps (do both legs together)	2	5 Minutes
	3-way Pendulum Legs with Chair support	10 each side	1	
	Hip Flexor Stretch	10 each side	2	
Main Workout	Banded Clamshells	10 up & down and 10 count holds (both sides)	3	17 Minutes
	Banded Glute Bridges	12 up & down and 10 count holds	3	
	Standing Banded Lateral Leg raises (Chair/wall supported)	12 each leg	3	
	Knee down, Side Plank	30 seconds each side	2	
Heart raisers	High Knees with Slow Jogging	30 seconds work, 15 seconds rest	2	3 Minutes
	Butt Kicks	30 seconds work, 15 seconds rest	2	
Stretching	Lying down Glute Stretch	20 seconds hold each side	2	5 Minutes
	Lying down Knee Hug	20 seconds hold	2	
	Seated Forward Bend	20 seconds hold	2	

Month 4, Week 1-4, Day 3 – Upper Body (Mini Band/Loop Band Workout)

Please scan this QR code for the YouTube Video

Group	Exercise	No. of Reps	No. of Sets	Time Required to Perform
Warm-Up	Small Arm Circles - Clockwise & Anticlockwise (quick ones)	10 each side	2	5-6 Minutes
	Overhead Back Touches	10 each side	2	
	Shoulder Touches	10 each side	2	
Main workout	Banded Wall Pushup	10	3	17 Minutes
	Banded Single-arm Triceps extension	10 each side	3	
	Banded Seated Single-arm, Bicep Curl	10 each side	3	
	Lying down, Leg Raises	15	3	
Heart raisers	Step Up & Down (stepper or 1st step of a staircase)	30 seconds work, 15 seconds rest	2	3 Minutes
	Jumping Jacks	30 seconds work, 15 seconds rest	2	
Stretching	Standing Triceps Stretch	20 seconds hold each side	2	5 Minutes
	Standing Arm Stretch	20 seconds hold each side	2	
	Wall Assisted Chest Stretch	20 seconds hold each side	2	

Month 4, Week 1-4, Day 4 – Lower Body (Mini Band/Loop Band Workout)

Please scan this QR code for the YouTube Video

Group	Exercise	No. of Reps	No. of Sets	Time Required to Perform
Warm-Up	Standing Butt kicks (Chair/wall Support) - Quick Movements	10 each leg	2	5 Minutes
	Seated BW Single-leg Extension	10 each + 10 both legs	1	
	Standing Hip Openers	10 each leg	2	
Main Workout	Banded seated Knee marches	10	3	17 Minutes
	Banded Air Squats	10	3	
	Banded single-leg Romanian Deadlift	10 each leg	3	
	3-way Heel raises	10 each way	3	
	Lying down Toe Taps	12 total (6 each leg)	2	
Heart Raisers	Side-to-side Shuffle	30 seconds work, 15 seconds rest	2	3 Minutes
	On-the-spot Jogging	30 seconds work, 15 seconds rest	2	
Stretching	Standing Quad Stretch	20 seconds hold each side	2	5 Minutes
	Standing IT Band Stretch	20 seconds hold each side	1	
	Standing Calf Stretch	20 seconds hold each side	2	

Month 5, Week 1-4, Day 1 – Upper Body (Bamboo Stick Mobility, Dumbbells and Ankle Weight Workout)

Please scan this QR code for the YouTube Video

Group	Exercise	No. of Reps	No. of Sets	Time Required to Perform
Warm-Up	Bamboo Stick Lat pulldown	12	2	6 Minutes
	Hip Hinged Y's and O's	12 each	2	
	Bamboo Stick Bicep Curl	12	2	
	Bamboo Stick Toe Touch and up	12	1	
Main Workout	DB single-arm Rowing (increase the weight)	12 each side	3	17 Minutes
	DB Upright Rows (increase the weight)	12	3	
	DB Bent Over Rows	12	3	
	DB Hammer Curl	12 total (6 each side)	3	
	High Plank	20 seconds hold	2	
Heart Raisers	Burpees (scale down version)	30 seconds work, 15 seconds rest	2	3 Minutes
	Grapevine	30 seconds work, 15 seconds rest	2	
Stretching	Wall-assisted Lat stretch	20 seconds hold	2	4 Minutes
	Twisted Yoga Pose	20 seconds hold each side	1	
	Arm Stretch	20 seconds hold each side	2	

Month 5, Week 1-4, Day 2 – Lower Body (Bamboo Stick Mobility, Dumbbells and Ankle Weight Workout)

Please scan this QR code for the YouTube Video

Group	Exercise	No. of Reps	No. of Sets	Time Required to Perform
Warm-Up	Quadruped Cat Camel	12	2	5 Minutes
	Dynamic Quad Stretch	10 each side	1	
	Hamstring Swipes	10 each side	2	
	Bamboo Stick Good Mornings	10	2	
Main Workout	Ankle Weight Seated Leg Extension (raise the height with Pillows)	10 each leg	3	18 Minutes
	Ankle Weight Donkey kicks (3 variations)	10 each leg (any variation that you are comfortable)	3	
	Ankle Weight Standing Lateral leg raises	10 each leg	3	
	Ankle Weight Lying Down Hamstring Curl	12	2	
	Beast Hold	20 seconds hold	2	
Heart Raisers	High Knees	30 seconds work, 15 seconds rest	2	3 Minutes
	Butt Kicks	30 seconds work, 15 seconds rest	2	
Stretching	Standing Quad Stretch	20 seconds hold each side	2	4 Minutes
	Standing Hamstring Stretch	20 seconds hold each side	2	

Month 5, Week 1-4, Day 3 – Upper Body (Bamboo Stick Mobility, Dumbbells and Ankle Weight Workout)

Please scan this QR code for the YouTube Video

Group	Exercise	No. of Reps	No. of Sets	Time Required to Perform
Warm-Up	Bamboo Stick Shoulder Dislocates	10	1	5 Minutes
	Bamboo Stick Front Raise to Overhead Press	12	2	
	Overhead Back Touches	12 each hand	2	
Main workout	DB Front Chest Press (increase the weight)	12	3	18 Minutes
	Seated DB Arnold Press	10	3	
	Standing DB Around the World	10	2	
	DB Triceps Overhead Extension (increase the weight)	10	3	
	Bamboo Stick Overhead side bending	16	3	
Heart Raisers	Jumping Jacks	30 seconds work, 15 seconds rest	2	3 Minutes
	Foot Fire	30 seconds work, 15 seconds rest	2	
Stretching	Standing Shoulder Stretch	20 seconds hold each side	2	4 Minutes
	Standing Triceps Stretch	20 seconds hold each side	1	
	Wall-assisted Chest Stretch	20 seconds hold each side	1	

Month 5, Week 1-4, Day 4 – Lower Body (Bamboo Stick Mobility, Dumbbells and Ankle Weight Workout)

Please scan this QR code for the YouTube Video

Group	Exercise	No. of Reps	No. of Sets	Time Required to Perform
Warm-Up	Mountain to Cobra	10	2	4 Minutes
	Hip Flexor Stretch	10 each side	1	
	Seated Heel Raises	15	1	
Main Workout	Ankle Weight Quadruped Fire Hydrant	10 each side	2	20 Minutes
	Ankle Weight Hurdle Crossing	10 each side	3	
	Seated Ankle Weight Heel Raises	15	3	
	Standing Ankle Weight Glute Kickback	8 each side (finish 1 side and then go with the other side)	3	
	Russian Twists	20	2	
Heart raisers	Standing Crunches (increase speed) (can wear ankle weights for making it challenging)	30 seconds work, 15 seconds rest	2	3 Minutes
	On-the-spot Jogging (can wear ankle weights for making it challenging)	30 seconds work, 15 seconds rest	2	
Stretching	Standing Glute Stretch	20 seconds hold each side	2	3 Minutes
	Standing Calf Stretch	20 seconds hold each side	1	

Month 6, Week 1-4, Day 1 – Lower Body (Resistance Band & Pilates Band Workout)

Please scan this QR code for the YouTube Video

Group	Exercise	No. of Reps	No. of Sets	Time Required to Perform
Warm-Up	Quadruped Cat Camel	12	2	4 Minutes
	Dynamic Quad Stretch	12 each leg	2	
	Hip Flexor Stretch	12 each leg	1	
Main Workout	Pilates Band Seated Leg Press	10 each leg	3	20 Minutes
	Resistance Band Deadlift	12	3	
	Resistance band Front Rack Chair Squats	10	3	
	BW Side Lunges	8 each side	2	
	Deadbug opposite Limb Movement	20	2	
Heart Raisers	Foot Fire	30 seconds work, 15 seconds rest	2	3 Minutes
	Butt Kicks with slow Jogging	30 seconds work, 15 seconds rest	2	
Stretching	Standing Quad Stretch	20 seconds hold each leg	1	3 Minutes
	Lying down Single Knee Hugs	20 seconds hold each leg	1	
	Pigeon Stretch	20 seconds hold each leg	1	

Month 6, Week 1-4, Day 2 – Upper Body (Resistance Band & Pilates Band Workout)

Please scan this QR code for the YouTube Video

Group	Exercise	No. of Reps	No. of Sets	Time Required to Perform
Warm-Up	Big Arm Circles - Forward & Backward	10 each way	2	4 Minutes
	Chest Stretch to Shoulder Stretch	10 each hand	1	
	OH, Back Touches	10 each hand	2	
Main workout	Resistance Band No money (Rotator cuff)	12	2	20 Minutes
	Resistance Band seated Shoulder Press	12 each hand	3	
	Resistance Band lying down Chest Press	12	3	
	Resistance Band OH Triceps Extension	12 each hand	3	
	Bicycle Crunches	20	2	
Heart Raisers	Step up (increase the speed)	30 seconds work, 15 seconds rest	2	3 Minutes
	Skipping/Jump Rope	30 seconds work, 15 seconds rest	2	
Stretching	Standing Shoulder Stretch	20 seconds hold each hand	1	2 Minutes
	Wall-assisted Chest Stretch	20 seconds hold each hand	1	
	Standing Triceps Stretch	20 seconds hold each hand	1	

Month 6, Week 1-4, Day 3 – Lower Body (Resistance Band & Pilates Band Workout)

Please scan this QR code for the YouTube Video

Group	Exercise	No. of Reps	No. of Sets	Time Required to Perform
Warm-Up	Mountain to Cobra	10	1	4 Minutes
	Bamboo Stick Good Mornings	12	2	
	Lateral Hip Flexor Stretch	10 each side	1	
Main workout	BW Quadruped Kickback	10 each leg	3	20 Minutes
	Pilates Band Lying down lateral side Press	10 each leg	3	
	Pilates Band Lying Down one leg Circles (clockwise and anticlockwise)	10 each leg	3	
	BW Quadruped hamstring Curl	10 each leg	2	
	Russian Twists	20	2	
Heart Raisers	Jumping Jacks	30 seconds work, 15 seconds rest	2	3 Minutes
	Zumba Dance Move	30 seconds work, 15 seconds rest	2	
Stretching	Lying Down Glute Stretch	20 seconds hold each leg	1	3 Minutes
	Standing IT Band stretch	20 seconds hold each side	1	

Month 6, Week 1-4, Day 4 – Upper Body (Resistance Band & Pilates Band Workout)

Please scan this QR code for the YouTube Video

Group	Exercise	No. of Reps	No. of Sets	Time Required to Perform
Warm-Up	Lying down IYWTO	10	1	4 Minutes
	Quadruped T Spine Rotation to Thread the Needle	10 each side	2	
	Shoulder Touches	12 each side	2	
Main workout	Pilates Band standing Lat Pulldown	15	3	20 Minutes
	Front Raise Band Pull apart	12	2	
	Resistance Band Seated Rowing	15	3	
	Resistance Band Bicep Curl	12	3	
	High Plank Toe Taps	12	2	
Heart raisers	DB (lightweight) Punches with Toe Taps (increase speed)	30 seconds work, 15 seconds rest	2	3 Minutes
	Side-to-side shuffle	30 seconds work, 15 seconds rest	2	
Stretching	Wall Assisted Lat Stretch	20 seconds hold	1	3 Minutes
	Supine Spine Twist	20 seconds hold each side	1	
	Standing Arm Stretch	20 seconds hold each side	1	

100

Month 7, Week 1-4, Day 1 – Lower Body (Dumbbells/Body Weight /Ankle Weights/Loop Bands/Bamboo Stick Workout)

Please scan this QR code for the YouTube Video

Group	Exercise	No. of Reps	No. of Sets	Time Required to Perform
Warm-Up	Quadruped Cat Camel	15	2	5 Minutes
	Hamstring Swipes	10 each side	1	
	Standing Hip Openers	10 each side	1	
Main Workout	DB Hip Thrusts with the Chair (increase the weight)	12	3	17 Minutes
	Wall Sit holds	45 seconds	2	
	Ankle Weight Quadruped Hamstring Curl (Single-leg)	10 each leg	3	
	Standing Heel raises	20	3	
	Mountain Climbers	20 (10 each leg)	2	
Heart Raisers	Foot Fire	30 seconds work, 15 seconds rest	2	3 Minutes
	Step up (increase the speed)	30 seconds work, 15 seconds rest	2	
Stretching	Standing Quad Stretch	20 seconds hold each leg	2	4 Minutes
	Standing Calf Stretch	20 seconds hold each leg	1	
	Lying Down Glute Stretch	20 seconds hold each leg	2	

Month 7, Week 1-4, Day 2 – Upper Body (Dumbbells/Body Weight /Ankle Weights/Loop Bands/Bamboo Stick Workout)

Please scan this QR code for the YouTube Video

Group	Exercise	No. of Reps	No. of Sets	Time Required to Perform
Warm-Up	Quadruped T spine Rotation to Thread the Needle	10 each side	2	5 Minutes
	Small Arm Circles - Clockwise & Anti Clockwise	10 each side	2	
	Dynamic Chest Stretch to Shoulder Stretch	20	1	
Main Workout	DB Lateral Raise to Front Raise	12	3	18 Minutes
	DB Chest Fly's	12	3	
	DB Single-arm Rowing	12 each side	3	
	Superman (hold for 2 seconds in each rep)	10	2	
	Deadbug Limb Extension	20	3	
Heart Raisers	On-the-spot Jogging	30 seconds work, 15 seconds rest	2	3 Minutes
	DB (lightweight) Punches with Toe Taps (increase speed)	30 seconds work, 15 seconds rest	2	
Stretching	Standing Shoulder Stretch	20 seconds hold each hand	1	4 Minutes
	Wall Assisted Lat stretch	20 seconds hold	1	
	Supine Spine Twist	20 seconds hold each side	2	

Month 7, Week 1-4, Day 3 – Lower Body (Dumbbells/Body Weight /Ankle Weights/Loop Bands/Bamboo Stick Workout)

Please scan this QR code for the YouTube Video

Group	Exercise	No. of Reps	No. of Sets	Time Required to Perform
Warm-Up	Mountain to Cobra	10	1	3 Minutes
	Seated 90-90 Hip Openers	10	1	
	Dynamic Quad Stretch	10 each leg	1	
Main Workout	Banded Clamshells	12 each side	3	20 Minutes
	DB Sumo Squats	12	3	
	Feet Elevated Glute Bridges (hamstring focused)	12	3	
	Ankle Weight Seated Leg Extension (raise the height with Pillows)	12 each leg	3	
	Bamboo Stick OH Side Bends	12	3	
Heart Raisers	Zumba Dance Move	30 seconds work, 15 seconds rest	2	3 Minutes
	Plank Jacks/ Plank Toe Taps	30 seconds work, 15 seconds rest	2	
Stretching	Standing Hamstring Stretch	20 seconds hold each side	1	3 Minutes
	Standing Quad Stretch	20 seconds hold each side	1	
	Pigeon Stretch/ Lying down Glute Stretch	20 seconds hold each side	1	

Month 7, Week 1-4, Day 4 – Upper Body (Dumbbells/Body Weight /Ankle Weights/Loop Bands/Bamboo Stick Workout)

Please scan this QR code for the YouTube Video

Group	Exercise	No. of Reps	No. of Sets	Time Required to Perform
Warm-Up	OH, Back Touches	10 each hand	2	5 Minutes
	Shoulder Touches	12 each hand	2	
	Bamboo Stick Shoulder Dislocates	10	1	
Main Workout	DB Triceps Kickback	12	3	18 Minutes
	Bench Dips/ DB Triceps OH Extension	10	3	
	DB Zottman Curls	10	3	
	DB Hammer Curl	12 each side	3	
	Side Plank Holds	30 seconds hold each side	2	
Heart Raisers	High Knee March (Jog slightly to make it challenging)	30 seconds work, 15 seconds rest	2	3 Minutes
	Skipping/Jump Rope	30 seconds work, 15 seconds rest	2	
Stretching	Standing Triceps Stretch	20 seconds hold each side	1	3 Minutes
	Standing Arm Stretch	20 seconds hold each side	1	
	Side Neck Stretch	20 seconds hold each side	1	

Month 8, Week 1-4, Day 1 – Lower Body (Dumbbells/Body Weight /Ankle Weights/Resistance/Pilates Bands/Bamboo Stick/ kettlebell Workout)

Please scan this QR code for the YouTube Video

Group	Exercise	No. of Reps	No. of Sets	Time Required to Perform
Warm-Up	Standing Hip Openers	10 each leg	1	4 Minutes
	Hip Hinging with Bamboo Stick	12	2	
	Dynamic Quad Stretch	10 each leg	1	
Main Workout	Ankle Weight Seated Leg Extension (raise the height with Pillows)	12 each leg (finish 1 leg & then start other leg in each set)	3	20 Minutes
	Quad Rockers	8	2	
	Sumo Squat with Heel Raises	10	3	
	Heel elevated Goblet Squat	10	3	
	Lying down Heel Slides	10 each leg (do alternate)	3	
Heart Raisers	Stepper side-to-side Touch Down	30 seconds work, 15 seconds rest	2	3 Minutes
	Standing crunches with Slight jumping	30 seconds work, 15 seconds rest	2	
Stretching	Static Quad Stretch	30 seconds each leg	1	3 Minutes
	Seated Ankle Stretch	20 seconds	1	
	Static Side bend Stretch	20 seconds each side	1	

Month 8, Week 1-4, Day 2 – Upper Body (Dumbbells/Body Weight /Ankle Weights/Resistance/Pilates Bands/Bamboo Stick/ kettlebell Workout)

Please scan this QR code for the YouTube Video

Group	Exercise	No. of Reps	No. of Sets	Time Required to Perform
Warm-Up	Hip-Hinged Y's & T's	10 Y's & 10T's	1	4 Minutes
	Quadruped T Spine Rotation to Thread the Needle	10 each side	1	
	Banded Pull Apart	12	2	
Main Workout	DB Shrugs	15	3	20 Minutes
	DB Single-arm Rowing	12 each hand	3	
	DB Deadlift (use at least 5 Kg DB)	10	3	
	Kettlebell/DB Swings	10	2	
	Bamboo Stick Deadbug Leg Extension	16	2	
Heart Raisers	On-the-spot Jogging (Increase the speed)	30 seconds work, 15 seconds rest	2	2 Minutes
	Jumping Jacks	30 seconds work, 15 seconds rest	2	
Stretching	Static Thread the Needle Stretch	20 seconds each side	1	3 Minutes
	Child's Pose hold	20 seconds hold	1	
	Lying down, Single-leg Knee Hug hold	20 seconds hold	1	

Month 8, Week 1-4, Day 3 – Lower Body (Dumbbells/Body Weight /Ankle Weights/Resistance/Pilates Bands/Bamboo Stick/ kettlebell Workout)

Please scan this QR code for the YouTube Video

Group	Exercise	No. of Reps	No. of Sets	Time Required to Perform
Warm-Up	Quadruped Cat Camel	10	2	4 Minutes
	Mountain Pose Marching	10 each leg	2	
	Hip Flexor Stretch	10 each leg	1	
Main Workout	DB Hip Thrusts with a Chair	15	3	20 Minutes
	Ankle Weight Standing Kickback	12 each leg	3	
	Foot Elevated Single-leg Hip Thrusts	10 ach leg	3	
	DB Romanian Deadlift (RDL)	12	3	
	Bicycle Crunches	20	2	
Heart Raisers	Foot Fire	30 seconds work, 15 seconds rest	2	2 Minutes
	Side-to-side Shuffle	30 seconds work, 15 seconds rest	2	
Stretching	Lying Down Glute Stretch	20 seconds hold each leg	1	3 Minutes
	Seated Forward bending	20 seconds hold	1	
	Butterfly Pose Hold	20 seconds hold	1	

Month 8, Week 1-4, Day 4 – Upper Body (Dumbbells/Body Weight /Ankle Weights/Resistance/Pilates Bands/Bamboo Stick/ kettlebell Workout)

Please scan this QR code for the YouTube Video

Group	Exercise	No. of Reps	No. of Sets	Time Required to Perform
Warm-Up	Bamboo Stick Shoulder Dislocates	10	1	4 Minutes
	Chest Stretch to Shoulder Stretch	12	1	
	OH, Back Touches	12	2	
Main Workout	DB Lying Down Chest Press	12	3	20 Minutes
	DB Arnold Press	10	3	
	DB Front Raise to Lateral Raise	10	3	
	Triceps Kick Back superset with the next exercise	10 (finish 10 reps of Kick back and without taking a break, immediately start Bench dips and complete 10 reps and then take a break)	3	
	Bench/Chair Dips			
Heart Raisers	Plank Toe Taps/Plank Jacks (Advanced)	30 seconds work, 15 seconds rest	2	2 Minutes
	Skipping/Jump Rope	30 seconds work, 15 seconds rest	2	
Stretching	Standing Triceps Stretch	20 seconds hold each side	1	3 Minutes
	Standing Shoulder Stretch	20 seconds hold each side	1	
	Wall-assisted Chest Stretch	20 seconds hold	1	

Month 9, Week 1-4, Day 1 – Upper Body (Dumbbells, Mini/Loop band, Resistance Band (hold & Pulses) Workout)

Please scan this QR code for the YouTube Video

Group	Exercise	No. of Reps	No. of Sets	Time Required to Perform
Warm-Up	Lying down IYWTO	10	1	4 Minutes
	Quadruped T Spine Rotation	10 each side	1	
	Shoulder Touches	12 each side	2	
Main Workout	Banded Single-arm Lat pulldown	Complete 10 reps on 1 side, pull and hold the band for 10 counts, and then move to the other side	3	20 Minutes
	DB Single-arm Row (increase to 5 kg DB)	12 each side	3	
	DB Upright Rows (increase to 5 kg DB)	10	3	
	Banded Bicep Curls (Resistance band)	10	3	
	DB Farmer's March	20 Marches	3	
Heart Raisers	Pop Squats	30 seconds work, 15 seconds rest	2	3 Minutes
	On-the-Spot Jogging	30 seconds work, 15 seconds rest	2	
Stretching	Static Thread the Needle	20 seconds hold each side	1	3 Minutes
	Wall-assisted Lat Stretch	20 seconds hold	1	
	Seated Arm Stretch	20 seconds hold each side	1	

Month 9, Week 1-4, Day 2 – Lower Body (Dumbbells, Mini/Loop band, Resistance Band (hold & Pulses) Workout)

Please scan this QR code for the YouTube Video

Group	Exercise	No. of Reps	No. of Sets	Time Required to Perform
Warm-Up	Hip Rotation - Clockwise and Anticlockwise	12 each side	1	3 Minutes
	Lateral Single-leg Raises	12 each side	1	
	Front and Back swings	12 each side	1	
Main Workout	Mini Banded One leg lateral Hip Abduction followed by Pulses (on the Chair)	complete 10 reps on both legs and do 15 pulses	3	20 Minutes
	Banded Glute Bridges followed by hold and butterfly pulses	complete 12 reps of Bridges, hold for 10 counts in the bridge position, and then flap your legs for 12 reps	3	
	Heel-elevated single-leg Hip Bridges	10 each side	3	
	3-way Heel Raises	10 each way	3	
	Beast Hold	30 seconds hold	3	
Heart Raisers	Foot Fire	30 seconds work, 15 seconds rest	2	3 Minutes
	Zumba Dance Move	30 seconds work, 15 seconds rest	2	
Stretching	Lying down Glute Stretch	20 seconds hold each side	1	2 Minutes
	Standing Calf Stretch	20 seconds hold each side	1	

Month 9, Week 1-4, Day 3 – Upper Body (Dumbbells, Mini/Loop band, Resistance Band (hold & Pulses) Workout)

Please scan this QR code for the YouTube Video

Group	Exercise	No. of Reps	No. of Sets	Time Required to Perform
Warm-Up	Resistance Band Shoulder Dislocates	10	1	4 Minutes
	Small Arm Circles - Clockwise & Anticlockwise followed by BW Shoulder Press	12 each of it	2	
	OH, Back Touches	15 each hand	2	
Main Workout	DB OH Press	12	3	20 Minutes
	DB Lateral Raise followed by Banded Lateral Raise (superset)	complete 8 DB reps and followed by 8 reps with band	3	
	Lying Down DB Chest Press followed by Banded Chest Flys (superset)	complete 8 DB reps and followed by 8 reps with band	3	
	DB Triceps kickback followed by Banded Triceps Extension (superset)	complete 8 DB reps and followed by 8 reps with band	3	
	Tabletop Crunches	15	3	
Heart Raisers	Side-to-side Shuffle	30 seconds work, 15 seconds rest	2	3 Minutes
	Step up (stepper)	30 seconds work, 15 seconds rest	2	
Stretching	Seated Shoulder Stretch	20 seconds hold each side	1	3 Minutes
	Standing Triceps Stretch	20 seconds hold each side	1	
	Wall-assisted Chest Stretch	20 Seconds hold	1	

Month 9, Week 1-4, Day 4 – Lower Body (Dumbbells, Mini/Loop band, Resistance Band (hold & Pulses) Workout)

Please scan this QR code for the YouTube Video

Group	Exercise	No. of Reps	No. of Sets	Time Required to Perform
Warm-Up	Dynamic Quad Stretch	12 each leg	1	3 Minutes
	BW Seated Leg Extension	15	2	
	Seated 90-90 Hip Openers	10	1	
Main Workout	DB Sumo Squat followed by BW Pulses	12 full squats and then 10 pulses	3	20 Minutes
	Mini Banded Squats with Lateral Leg Raise	12	3	
	BW Side Lunges	12	3	
	DB Goblet Squat (increase to 5 kg DB)	12	3	
	Plank Shoulder Taps	30 seconds	2	
Heart Raisers	Grapevine	30 seconds work, 15 seconds rest	2	3 Minutes
	Stepper side-to-side touch-down	30 seconds work, 15 seconds rest	2	
Stretching	Standing Quad Stretch	20 seconds hold each side	1	3 Minutes
	Seated Adductor Stretch (wide-legged forward bend)	20 Seconds hold	1	
	Sphinx Pose	20 seconds hold each side	1	

Month 10, Week 1-4, Day 1 – Full Body (Dumbbells & Resistance Band mix Workout)

Please scan this QR code for the YouTube Video

Group	Exercise	No. of Reps	No. of Sets	Time Required to Perform
Warm-Up	Quadruped Cat Camel	12	2	4 Minutes
	Hip Flexor Stretch	12	1	
	World's Greatest Stretch	8 each side	1	
Main Workout	Squat Thrusters	10	3	20 Minutes
	Single-leg Glute Bridge (2 ways to be done in the video; you can choose any one of the ways that you are comfortable)	10 each side	3	
	DB Chest fly's	10	3	
	Resistance Band Bent over Rows	12	3	
	Plank to toe Touch	30 seconds	2	
Heart Raisers	Stepper side-to-side touch-down	45 seconds work 15 seconds rest	1	2 Minutes
	Pop Squats	45 seconds work 15 seconds rest	1	
Stretching	Standing Quad Stretch	20 seconds each side	1	3 Minutes
	Thread the Needle	20 seconds each side	1	
	Twisted Yoga Pose	20 seconds each side	1	

113

Month 10, Week 1-4, Day 2 – Full Body (Dumbbells & Resistance Band mix Workout)

Please scan this QR code for the YouTube Video

Group	Exercise	No. of Reps	No. of Sets	Time Required to Perform
Warm-Up	Mountain to Cobra	10	1	3 Minutes
	Lying down IYWTO	10	1	
	Hamstring Swipes	10 each leg	1	
Main Workout	Single-leg DB Romanian Deadlift (with Chair Support)	12	2	20 Minutes
	Standing Banded Triceps Extension	12	3	
	Resistance band Lat pull down	12	3	
	DB Bicep Curl	12	3	
	Inch Worm to Shoulder Taps	10	2	
Heart Raisers	Skipping/Jump Rope	45 seconds work 15 seconds rest	1	2 Minutes
	Standing Crunch with Jumping	45 seconds work 15 seconds rest	1	
Stretching	Lying down Hamstring Stretch with resistance band	20 seconds each side	1	3 Minutes
	Puppy dog Pose	20 seconds hold	1	
	Standing Triceps Stretch	20 seconds each side	1	

Month 10, Week 1-4, Day 3 – Full Body (Dumbbells & Resistance Band mix Workout)

Please scan this QR code for the YouTube Video

Group	Exercise	No. of Reps	No. of Sets	Time Required to Perform
Warm-Up	3-way Neck stretch	10 each	1	4 Minutes
	Hip Rotation - Clockwise & Anticlockwise	10 each side	2	
	Bamboo Stick Good Mornings	12	1	
Main Workout	Butterfly Glute Bridges with heavy DB	15	3	20 Minutes
	Resistance band Upright Rows	12	3	
	Resistance Band Front squats	12	3	
	DB Shrugs (increase the weight to 5 KG DB)	15	3	
	Bird Dog	16	2	
Heart Raisers	Zumba Dance Move	45 seconds work 15 seconds rest	1	2 Minutes
	Step Touch with Hand Movement (use lightweight DB to make it challenging)	45 seconds work 15 seconds rest	1	
Stretching	Lying down Glute stretch	20 seconds each side	1	3 Minutes
	Standing Quad stretch	20 seconds each side	1	
	Standing Shoulder Stretch	20 seconds each side	1	

Month 10, Week 1-4, Day 4 – Full Body (Dumbbells & Resistance Band mix Workout)

Please scan this QR code for the YouTube Video

Group	Exercise	No. of Reps	No. of Sets	Time Required to Perform
Warm-Up	Standing Ankle Rotation Clockwise & Anticlockwise	10 each side, each leg	1	3 Minutes
	Chest Stretch to Shoulder Stretch	10	1	
	Mountain to Cobra	10	1	
Main Workout	DB Chest Press	12	3	20 Minutes
	DB Lateral Raise to Front Raise	12	3	
	Db Swings (use at least 4 kg DB)	10	3	
	DB 3-way Heel Raises	10 each way	3	
	Crunches with Punches	12	2	
Heart Raisers	Jumping Jack	45 seconds work 15 seconds rest	1	2 Minutes
	Mountain Climbers	45 seconds work 15 seconds rest	1	
Stretching	Standing Shoulder Stretch	20 seconds each side	1	3 Minutes
	Standing Calf Stretch	20 seconds each side	1	
	Sphinx Pose	30 seconds hold	1	

Month 11, Week 1-4, Day 1 – Lower Body (Dumbbells & Body Weight Workout) – Advanced

Please scan this QR code for the YouTube Video

Group	Exercise	No. of Reps	No. of Sets	Time Required to Perform
Warm-Up	Mountain to Cobra	10	1	3 Minutes
	Hamstring Swipes	10 each leg	1	
	Lateral Hip Flexor Stretch	10 each leg	1	
Main Workout	Step up on the Chair	10 each leg	2	17 Minutes
	BW Reverse Lunge with Chair Support	10 each leg	2	
	DB Romanian Deadlift (increase the weight to 5KG DB or more)	12	3	
	DB Sumo Squat	12	3	
	Banded Mountain Climber Holds	8 each leg (5 count holds)	2	
Heart Raisers	Foot Fire	45 seconds work 15 seconds rest	1	2 Minutes
	High Knees Jogging	45 seconds work 15 seconds rest	1	
Stretching	Lying Down Single-leg Knee Hug	20 seconds each leg	2	5 Minutes
	Butterfly Stretch	20 seconds hold	2	
	Lying down Hamstring Stretch with Resistance band	20 seconds each leg	2	

Month 11, Week 1-4, Day 2 – Upper Body (Dumbbells & Body Weight Workout) – Advanced

Please scan this QR code for the YouTube Video

Group	Exercise	No. of Reps	No. of Sets	Time Required to Perform
Warm-Up	BW Shoulder Press	12	2	4 Minutes
	World's Greatest Stretch	8 each side	1	
	Bamboo Stick Shoulder Dislocates	10	1	
Main Workout	DB Arnold Press (increase the DB weight)	12	3	20 Minutes
	DB Around the world	12	2	
	DB Chest Flys	12	3	
	DB Skull Crushers	10	3	
	Bench Dips	10	3	
Heart Raisers	Standing crunches with Jumping	45 seconds work 15 seconds rest	1	2 Minutes
	Stepper side-to-side touch-down	45 seconds work 15 seconds rest	1	
Stretching	Standing Shoulder Stretch	20 seconds each leg	1	3 Minutes
	Wall-assisted Chest Stretch	20 seconds each leg	1	
	Standing Triceps Stretch	20 seconds each leg	1	

Month 11, Week 1-4, Day 3 – Lower Body (Dumbbells & Body Weight Workout) – Advanced

Please scan this QR code for the YouTube Video

Group	Exercise	No. of Reps	No. of Sets	Time Required to Perform
Warm-Up	Dynamic Quad Stretch	10 each leg	1	4 Minutes
	Quadruped Cat Camel	10	2	
	Toe Hold Squat	10	1	
Main Workout	DB Front Squats (increase DB weight)	12	3	17 Minutes
	Sumo Squat with Heel Raises	12	3	
	Quad Rockers	12	2	
	Single-leg Heel Raises	10 each leg	3	
	Balance Chop	20	2	
Heart Raisers	Step Up & down on Stepper (increase the speed)	45 seconds work 15 seconds rest	1	2 Minutes
	Grapevine	45 seconds work 15 seconds rest	1	
Stretching	Static Quad Stretch	20 seconds hold each side	1	5 Minutes
	Pigeon Stretch	20 seconds hold each side	2	
	Standing Calf Stretch	20 seconds hold each side	1	

Month 11, Week 1-4, Day 4 – Upper Body (Dumbbells & Body Weight Workout) – Advanced

Please scan this QR code for the YouTube Video

Group	Exercise	No. of Reps	No. of Sets	Time Required to Perform
Warm-Up	Hip-Hinged Y's and T's	10 each	1	4 Minutes
	Band Pull Apart	10	2	
	Bent over Twist	15	1	
Main Workout	DB Deadlift (increase weight to 5KG or more)	12	3	20 Minutes
	DB Single-arm Rowing (increase weight to 5KG or more)	12 each side	3	
	DB Swings	12	3	
	DB Hammer Curl (increase the weight)	12	3	
	Side Plank Holds	30 seconds each side	2	
Heart Raisers	Jumping Jacks	45 seconds work 15 seconds rest	1	2 Minutes
	Plank Jacks	45 seconds work 15 seconds rest	1	
Stretching	Child's Pose Hold	20 seconds hold	1	3 Minutes
	Twisted Yoga Pose	20 seconds hold each side	1	
	Standing Arm Stretch	20 seconds hold each side	1	

Month 12, Week 1-4, Day 1 – Lower Body (Dumbbells & Body Weight Workout) – Advanced

Please scan this QR code for the YouTube Video

Group	Exercise	No. of Reps	No. of Sets	Time Required to Perform
Warm-up	Seated 90-90 Hip Openers	10	1	4 Minutes
	Hip Flexor Stretch	10 each leg	1	
	Air Squats	12	2	
Main Workout	Walking Lunges (hold DB to make it challenging)	walk at least 10 steps in each set	3	20 Minutes
	DB Front Rack squats followed by BW Pulses (use heavy DB)	12 full squats followed by 10 pulses	3	
	DB Step up on Chair	10 each leg	3	
	BW Sumo Squat to Lunge	10	2	
	Elbow Plank Holds	1 minute	1	
Heart Raisers	Burpees (Jumping)	45 seconds work 15 seconds rest	1	2 Minutes
	DB Floor to OH Press	45 seconds work 15 seconds rest	1	
Stretching	Standing Quad Stretch	20 seconds hold each leg	1	3 Minutes
	Seated Wide-legged forward bend (adductor stretch)	20 seconds hold	1	
	Pigeon Stretch	20 seconds hold each leg	1	

Month 12, Week 1-4, Day 2 – Upper Body (Dumbbells & Body Weight Workout) – Advanced

Group	Exercise	No. of Reps	No. of Sets	Time Required to Perform	QR code for Video
Warm-Up	Small Arm Circles - Clockwise & Anticlockwise followed by BW Shoulder Press	10 each	2	4 Minutes	
	Chest Stretch to Shoulder Stretch	10	1		
	Bamboo Stick Shoulder Dislocates	10	1		

Month 12, Week 1-4, Day 2 – Upper Body (Dumbbells & Body Weight Workout) – Advanced – Continuation

Group	Exercise	No. of Reps	No. of Sets	Time Required to Perform	QR code for Video
Main Workout	DB Arnold Press (drop set)	10 reps with heavier DB and then drop the weight, continue reps with lightest DB till failure	3	20 Minutes	
	DB Lateral Raise (drop set)	10 reps with heavier DB and then drop the weight, continue reps with lightest DB till failure	3		
	DB Chest Press followed by Chest Flys (superset)	use heavyweight - 8 reps of Chest Press immediately (without a break) followed by 8 reps of Chest Flys (Use Lightweight)	3		
	Skull Crushers Followed by Bench Dips (superset)	use Lightweight - 8 reps of Skull Crushers immediately (without a break) followed by 8 reps of Bench Dips	3		

123

Month 12, Week 1-4, Day 2 – Upper Body (Dumbbells & Body Weight Workout) – Advanced – Continuation

Group	Exercise	No. of Reps	No. of Sets	Time Required to Perform	QR code for Video
Heart Raisers	On-the-spot Jogging with Ankle Weights	45 seconds work 15 seconds rest	1	2 Minutes	
	Side-to-side shuffle	45 seconds work 15 seconds rest	1		
Stretching	Wall-assisted Chest Stretch	20 seconds hold each side	1	3 Minutes	
	Standing Shoulder Stretch	20 seconds hold each side	1		
	Standing Triceps Stretch	20 seconds hold each side	1		

Month 12, Week 1-4, Day 3 – Lower Body (Dumbbells & Body Weight Workout) – Advanced

Please scan this QR code for the YouTube Video

Group	Exercise	No. of Reps	No. of Sets	Time Required to Perform
Warm-up	BW Glute Bridges	15	1	4 Minutes
	Bamboo Stick Good Mornings	12	1	
	Lateral Hip Flexor Stretch	10 each side	1	
Main Workout	Courtesy Lunges/Bulgarian Split Squat (you can choose to do either one that you feel comfortable)	10 each leg	2	20 Minutes
	Banded Heel raised squat Hip Abduction	12	3	
	Heavy Weight Banded Hip thrusts	12	3	
	B Stance Romanian Deadlift	10 each leg	3	
	Single-leg foot Elevated Bridges (hamstring focused)	Complete 8 on 1 leg, do 8 on both legs and then do 8 on another leg without break	2	
Heart Raisers	Mountain Climbers	45 seconds work 15 seconds rest	1	2 Minutes
	Jumping Jacks	45 seconds work 15 seconds rest	1	
Stretching	Lying down Hamstring Stretch with Resistance Band	20 seconds hold each side	1	3 Minutes
	Lying down Glute Stretch	20 seconds hold each side	1	
	Supine Spine Twist	20 seconds hold each side	1	

125

Month 12, Week 1-4, Day 4 – Upper Body (Dumbbells & Body Weight Workout) – Advanced

Please scan this QR code for the YouTube Video

Group	Exercise	No. of Reps	No. of Sets	Time Required to Perform
Warm-up	Lying Down IYWTO	10	1	4 Minutes
	Mountain to cobra	10	1	
	Bamboo Stick Deadbug Leg Extension	8 each leg	2	
Main Workout	Heavy DB Deadlift	12	3	20 Minutes
	DB Bent over Rowing	10	3	
	Resistance Band Lat Pull Down	15	3	
	DB/KB Swings	12	3	
	Leg Tuckins	20	2	
Heart Raisers	High Knees	45 seconds work 15 seconds rest	1	2 Minutes
	Russian Twists	45 seconds work 15 seconds rest	1	
Stretching	Twisted Yoga Pose	20 seconds hold each side	1	3 Minutes
	Child's Pose	20 seconds hold	1	
	Sphinx Pose	20 seconds hold	1	

High-Intensity Interval Training (HIIT)

HIIT involves short bursts of strong exercise followed by rest periods, which boosts cardiovascular health, burns fat, and improves endurance.

Like all other workout programs, the YouTube videos for HIIT demonstrate only the exercises. You'll perform the exercises as written in the book.

- HIIT Programs: Six programs in total, with HIIT 1 to 3 for beginners and HIIT 4 to 6 for intermediate/advanced levels.
- Structure: Each HIIT program has four exercises - a combination of mostly bodyweight cardio and core exercises that need to be performed in a circuit manner.
- Warm-Up and Cool-Down: Always remember to warm up before starting HIIT and cool down after finishing. (You can use Month 1 Week 1's exercises for warm-up and stretching for cool down.)
- Timing: Perform each exercise for 30 seconds, followed by a 15-second break. Complete 3 to 4 rounds for best results. For example, If the HIIT program includes Jumping Jacks, Flutter Kicks, High Knees, and Plank to Toe Touch, perform 30 seconds of Jumping Jacks, take a 15-second break, then 30 seconds of Flutter Kicks, and so on. This completes one circuit. Aim to complete at least 3 to 4 circuits.

YouTube Support: There are YouTube videos with timers and music to help you keep track of the timing. See here:

https://www.youtube.com/watch?v=PzLaC3gkMUE

HIIT 1

Please scan this QR code for the YouTube Video

Exercise	Workout Time	Rest Time	Rounds
Jumping Jack	30 Seconds	15 Seconds	At least 3
Flutter Kicks	30 Seconds	15 Seconds	
High Knees	30 Seconds	15 Seconds	
Plank to Toe Touch	30 Seconds	15 Seconds	

HIIT 2

Please scan this QR code for the YouTube Video

Exercise	Workout Time	Rest Time	Rounds
Step up	30 Seconds	15 Seconds	At least 3
Lying Down Leg Raises	30 Seconds	15 Seconds	
Side-to-Side Shuffle	30 Seconds	15 Seconds	
Russian Twists	30 Seconds	15 Seconds	

HIIT 3

Please scan this QR code for the YouTube Video

Exercise	Workout Time	Rest Time	Rounds
High Knees	30 Seconds	15 Seconds	
Elbow plank to High Plank	30 Seconds	15 Seconds	At least 3
Burpee scale-down version	30 Seconds	15 Seconds	
Bird Dog	30 Seconds	15 Seconds	

HIIT 4

Please scan this QR code for the YouTube Video

Exercise	Workout Time	Rest Time	Rounds
Speed Skaters	45 Seconds	15 Seconds	
Renegade Rows	45 Seconds	15 Seconds	
DB Floor to OH Press	45 Seconds	15 Seconds	At least 3
Stepper Side-to-side Touch Down	45 Seconds	15 Seconds	

HIIT 5

Please scan this QR code for the YouTube Video

Exercise	Workout Time	Rest Time	Rounds
Plank Pike Jumps	30 Seconds	15 Seconds	At least 3
Banded leg Abduction Crunch	30 Seconds	15 Seconds	
Jumping Burpees	30 Seconds	15 Seconds	
Forward Lunge with a Twist	30 Seconds	15 Seconds	

HIIT 6

Please scan this QR code for the YouTube Video

Exercise	Workout Time	Rest Time	Rounds
Stepper Side-to-side Touch Down	30 Seconds	15 Seconds	At least 3
Side Lunge Twist	30 Seconds	15 Seconds	
High Knees	30 Seconds	15 Seconds	
DB Woodchopper	30 Seconds	15 Seconds	

Interactive Section: Reflecting On Your Workout Journey

1. Which of the ready-made plans have you tried?

2. How have the alternative exercises for floor work or the use of different equipment impacted your workout experience?

3. Get Competitive!

Encourage your friends and family to join you in a workout you enjoy. Make it a fun competition and tag the book and the publisher on social media with your progress and experiences.

4. Share Your Success Stories

We would love to hear about your fitness journey! Submit your success stories after following the workout plans. Highlight your progress and the impact on your fitness journey as a review.

DETAILED WORKOUT LOG

Use the following template to log your workouts. Monitoring your progress will motivate you and help you see how far you've come.

Date	Exercise	Weight (Lbs./kg)	Sets	Reps
1-Sep-2024	Shoulder Press	10 Lbs.	3	12

Feel free to make copies of this log or create your personalized version to keep track of your progress. Regularly updating your log will help you stay consistent and reach your fitness goals.

The next chapter is designed to diversify and intensify your workouts, leveraging the unique advantages that gym settings provide. Prepare to explore three months' worth of ready-made gym workout plans, made to fit a 30-minute-a-day, four-days-a-week schedule, just like your home routine but amplified with the variety and complexity that gym equipment offers.

CHAPTER SIX (BONUS)
Ready-Made Workout Programs At The Gym

Welcome to the bonus chapter you've been eagerly waiting for! In this section, we're introducing ready-made workout programs designed specifically for the gym. These programs are tailored to fit seamlessly into your lifestyle and require just 30 minutes a day, four days a week, for three months.

Whether you're a gym newbie or a seasoned regular, these structured plans will help you make the most of your gym time, maximizing your strength, flexibility, and overall fitness. Get ready to transform your gym experience and take your fitness journey to the next level!

Essential Instructions Before Starting Your Gym Workouts

Gym workouts can be started only after completing three months of home workouts.

There are QR codes linked to YouTube videos for all of the above exercise demonstrations. The videos demonstrate the correct form and technique only, so you won't be working out along with them. Instead, watch and learn the proper form, then perform the prescribed reps. This way, you can ensure you're doing each exercise correctly and safely, maximizing your results!

General Instructions

Before starting any workout, please do the following (now get up and look at yourself in the mirror and try the below instructions)

1. Engage Your Core:

Pull your navel to your spine. Imagine someone has tied a rope to your belly button and they are pulling it toward your spine to ensure you are engaging your core/abdominal muscles fully.

2. Keep Your Spine Straight

Give an anterior tilt to your pelvic girdle so that your spine is straight and there is no arching at your lower back.

3. Shoulders should always be retracted and depressed:

Roll back your shoulders and keep your shoulder blades together. Imagine you are pushing your shoulder blades into the back pockets of your jeans. This will ensure you are not hunching and are engaging your Lat muscles (side upper back muscles), protecting your spine when you lift heavy and in exercises that require bending forward.

4. Breathing:

Breathe in and out, and do not hold your breath during any exercises.

5. Incline Walks on the Treadmill:

Always hold the bar/support of the treadmill while doing incline walks, at least until you get used to the machine.

6. Setting Up Machines:

Always set up machines according to your height and safety. Check with a general trainer initially to understand the machine, then proceed.

Exercise-Specific Instructions

We've provided detailed instructions for a few key exercises that might be challenging to master just by watching a video. These exercises are crucial for building strength, improving form, and ensuring you get the most out of your workouts. While most of the exercises can be easily followed along with our YouTube videos, these specific ones require a bit more attention to technique and detail. Dive in, carefully read these instructions, and feel confident as you tackle these important movements. Remember, mastering these will set a solid foundation for your fitness journey!

Back Rack Squats:

- Always start with a small bar, placing the bar just below your Neck on your traps and not on your Neck.
- Squat on a bench until you get used to the weight
- You can use the big bar from the squat rack once you are used to the form as well as the weight
- In the YouTube video, I have shown how to start with a small bar and then move to a big bar and how to rack and un rack the big bar from the squat rack.
- You can also squat using smith machine to reap all the benefits of this powerful exercise.
- Stand up with your legs Hip-width apart, feet parallel to each other
- Naval pulled to spine
- Hinge your hip and go down as though you are sitting on a Chair, activating your quadriceps (front of your thighs)
- Ensure your Chest is up and not leaning too forward - imagine a big smiley on your t-shirt; when you squat, that smiley should be entirely visible.
- To begin with, go down as much as possible only; with practice, you can squat deeper.

Smith Machine Deadlift:

- Start with a plain bar and then add small weights and move up the weight as you get used to doing the correct form - the same is shown in the YouTube video
- Stand up with your legs Hip width apart, feet parallel to each other
- Naval pulled to spine - engage your core, pelvic tilted - neutral spine, shoulders retracted and depressed.

- Make sure you place your foot so that your shoelace is under the bar and your ankles are just Touching the bar.
- Now lean forward and hold the bar outside your foot, squat down with a neutral spine, keeping your upper back engaged, push through your heels, and straighten your hips, extending it fully and squeezing your glutes. The bar moves up along your legs and hips.

Barbell Hip Thrusts:

- Sit on the ground with your back against the bench (start with a decline bench, so it becomes easy to lean)
- Keep the barbell ready with big plates on the side, even though they weigh small, so you roll over the barbell towards you.
- Rest your upper back (just below your shoulder blades) on the bench
- Place your feet flat on the ground, shoulder-width apart, with your Knees bent.
- Naval Pulled to spine, push through your heels to lift your hips toward the ceiling.
- Lift your hips until your body is in a straight line from your Knees to your shoulders. Bend your Knees at 90 degrees at the top of the movement.
- At the top, squeeze your glutes (butt muscles) hard and hold for a moment.
- Slowly lower your hips back down to the ground, but do not let them Touch the ground completely. Keep the tension in your glutes.

Leg Press:

- The leg Press is a machine in the gym that works on different muscles of your legs.
- The foot placement differs for it to target these different muscles.
- Start by adjusting the machine for your height.

- For a quadriceps-focused leg Press, Step into the center of the platform with your foot hip-width apart, then bend your Knees so that your thighs get close to your Chest.
- Push through your heels to straighten your legs, ensuring you do not lock your Knees.
- Always start with 0 weights and then move up your weights
- For a glute and hamstring-focused leg Press, place your feet right on top of the platform, close to each other, about 1 to 1.5 inches apart, and repeat the above steps.

Reverse Lunge:
- Take a big step backward with your right foot.
- Bend both Knees to lower your body. Your right Knee should be just above the floor, and your left Knee should be at a 90-degree angle directly above your ankle.
- Maintain an Upright torso and keep your weight evenly distributed.
- Push through your left heel to return to the starting position, bringing your right foot forward.
- In the video, I have shown one leg going back into a lunge. However, the work is happening on the glutes/quads of the leg that is stationary.

Diversifying And Intensifying Your Workouts With Gym Equipment

Now, it's time to take your fitness journey to the next level. Leveraging gym equipment can help you diversify and intensify your workouts. This chapter includes a 3-month ready-made effective workout plan that seamlessly fits into your lifestyle, with just 30 minutes a day, four days a week.

What's Included in the Workout Plans
- Warm-Up: Essential to prepare your body for the workout.
- Targeted Muscle Exercises: Focus on different muscle groups using higher weights.

- Machines, Pulleys, and Other Equipment: Utilize various gym equipment for a comprehensive workout.
- Compound and Rotational Movements: Enhance strength, flexibility and balance.
- Core Strengthening and Stability: Build a strong and stable core.
- Cardiovascular Movements: Boost your heart health and endurance.

IMPORTANT: All exercises have QR codes linked to YouTube videos demonstrating them. The videos provide demonstrations only; follow the prescribed reps and sets as detailed in the workout program in this book.

The Gym Workout Programs

Month 1, Week 1-4, Day 1 (Lower Body)

Please scan this QR code for the YouTube Video

Group	Exercise	No. of Reps	No. of Sets	Time Required to Perform
Warm-Up	Standing Hip Openers	10 each leg	1	5 Minutes
	Air Squats/BW Squats	12	1	
	Hip Flexor Stretch	10 each leg	1	
	Quadruped Cat Camel	12	1	
Main workout	Deadbug Limb Extension	10 each side	1	15 Minutes
	Small Barbell Back Rack Squats	12	3	
	Leg Press Machine (start with no weight/light weight and gradually increase weight)	12	3	
	Leg Extension Machine (start with no weight/light weight and gradually increase weight)	12	3	
	Seated Calf Raises Machine (start with no weight/light weight and gradually increase weight)	10	3	
Cardio	Incline Treadmill Walk	NA	NA	8 Minutes
Stretching	Standing Quad Stretch	20 seconds each leg	1	2 Minutes
	Standing Calf Stretch	20 seconds each leg	1	

Month 1, Week 1-4, Day 2 (Upper Body)

Please scan this QR code for the YouTube Video

Group	Exercise	No. of Reps	No. of Sets	Time Required to Perform
Warm-Up	3-way Neck Stretch	10 each way	1	5 Minutes
	Shoulder Rotation - Forward & Backward	10 each side	2	
	Bamboo Stick OH Press	15	1	
	Bamboo Stick Shoulder Dislocates	10	1	
Main Workout	Shoulder Press Machine	10	3	15 Minutes
	DB Lateral Raise	12	3	
	Chest Press Machine	10	3	
	Cable Triceps Pushdown (bar Attached)	12	3	
	Beast Hold Shoulder Taps	30 seconds	2	
Cardio	Cross Trainer	NA	NA	8 Minutes
Stretching	Shoulder Stretch	20 seconds hold each side	1	2-3 Minutes
	Wall-assisted Chest Stretch	20 seconds hold	1	
	Triceps Stretch	20 seconds hold each side	1	

Month 1, Week 1-4, Day 3 (Lower Body)

Please scan this QR code for the YouTube Video

Group	Exercise	No. of Reps	No. of Sets	Time Required to Perform
Warm-Up	Mountain to Cobra	10	1	5 Minutes
	Bamboo Stick Good Mornings	10	1	
	BW Glute Bridges	15	1	
	Banded Clamshells	10 each side	1	
Main workout	Barbell Hip Thrusts (start with a small bar and low weights and use a decline bench)	12	3	15 Minutes
	DB Reverse Lunge (start with weight one size heavier than that you can EASILY lift)	8 each side	3	
	Smith Machine Romanian Deadlift (start with the plain bar and then slowly increase the weight)	12	3	
	Leg Curl Machine (start with no weight/light weight and gradually increase weight)	12	3	
	Bicycle Crunches	20	2	
Cardio	Incline Treadmill Walk	NA	NA	8 Minutes
Stretching	Lying down Glute Stretch	20 seconds each side	1	2-3 Minutes
	Hamstring Stretch with Resistance Band	20 seconds each side	1	

Month 1, Week 1-4, Day 4 (Upper Body)

Please scan this QR code for the YouTube Video

Group	Exercise	No. of Reps	No. of Sets	Time Required to Perform
Warm-Up	Resistance band Lat pull down	12	1	5 Minutes
	Child's Pose to Cobra	10	1	
	Lying Down IYWTO	10 IsYsWsTsOs	1	
	Quadruped T Spine Rotation	10 each side	1	
Main workout	Lat Pull Down Machine (start with no weight/light weight and gradually increase weight)	12	3	15 Minutes
	Cable Seated Rowing (start with no weight/light weight and gradually increase weight)	12	3	
	Hyper Extension Machine	8-10	3	
	Cable Bicep Curl (bar Attached) (start with no weight/light weight and gradually increase weight)	12	3	
	Russian Twists	20	2	
Cardio	Cross Trainer			8 Minutes
Stretching	Puppy Dog Pose	20 seconds hold	1	2-3 Minutes
	Arm Stretch	20 seconds hold each side	1	

Month 2, Week 1-4, Day 1 (Lower Body)

Please scan this QR code for the YouTube Video

Group	Exercise	No. of Reps	No. of Sets	Time Required to Perform
Warm-Up	Mountain to Cobra	10	1	5 Minutes
	Bamboo Stick Good Mornings	10	1	
	Banded Glute Bridges	12	1	
	Banded Lateral Walks	4 steps each side - 8 rounds	1	
Main Workout	Cable Romanian Deadlift	12	3	15 Minutes
	Foot Elevated Glute Bridges (hamstring-focused)	12	3	
	Barbell Hip Thrusts	12	3	
	DB Standing Calf raises	15	3	
	DB Deadbug Leg Extension	30 seconds	2	
Cardio	Incline Treadmill Walk	NA	NA	8 Minutes
Stretching	Lying Down Glute Stretch	20 seconds hold each side	1	2-3 Minutes
	Seated Forward Bending	20 seconds hold	1	
	Standing Calf Stretch	20 seconds hold each side	1	

Month 2, Week 1-4, Day 2 (Upper Body)

Please scan this QR code for the YouTube Video

Group	Exercise	No. of Reps	No. of Sets	Time Required to Perform
Warm-Up	Small Arm Circles - Clockwise and Anticlockwise to BW Shoulder Press	12 each side	1	5 Minutes
	Resistance Band Shoulder Dislocates	10	1	
	Resistance Band Dynamic Chest Stretch	10	1	
	Dynamic Triceps Stretch	10	1	
Main workout	Chest Fly Machine	12	3	15 Minutes
	Seated DB Shoulder Press	12	3	
	Cable Triceps Push Down (Bar Attached)	12	3	
	DB Triceps Kickback	12	3	
	Side Plank Holds	30 seconds	2	
Cardio	Incline Treadmill Walk	NA	NA	8 Minutes
Stretching	Thread the Needle holds	20 seconds hold each side	1	2-3 Minutes
	Wall-assisted Chest Stretch	20 seconds hold	1	
	Triceps Stretch	20 seconds hold each side		

Month 2, Week 1-4, Day 3 (Lower Body)

Please scan this QR code for the YouTube Video

Group	Exercise	No. of Reps	No. of Sets	Time Required to Perform
Warm-Up	Seated 90-90 Hip openers	10	1	5 Minutes
	Quadruped Cat Camel	12	1	
	Air Squats/BW Squats	12	1	
	Lateral Hip Flexor Stretch	10 each side	1	
Main workout	Heel Elevated Goblet Squats	12	3	15 Minutes
	Leg Press Machine	12	3	
	Leg Extension Machine	12	3	
	DB Sumo Squat	12	3	
	Lying Down, Leg raises	12	3	
Cardio	Incline Treadmill Walk	NA	NA	8 Minutes
Stretching	Standing Quad Stretch	20 seconds hold each side	1	2-3 Minutes
	Wide-legged Seated forward bend	20 seconds hold	1	

Month 2, Week 1-4, Day 4 (Upper Body)

Please scan this QR code for the YouTube Video

Group	Exercise	No. of Reps	No. of Sets	Time Required to Perform
Warm-Up	3-way Neck Stretch	10 each way	1	5 Minutes
	World's Greatest Stretch	10 each side	1	
	Lying down IYWTO	10 IsYsWsTsOs	1	
	Superman	10	1	
Main workout	Assisted Pull up (machine)	12	3	15 Minutes
	Wide grip Cable Lat pull down	12	3	
	Smith Machine Deadlift	10	3	
	Barbell Bicep Curl	10	3	
	DB Side Bending	12 each side	3	
Cardio	Incline Treadmill Walk	NA	NA	8 Minutes
Stretching	Machine-assisted Lat Stretch	20 seconds hold	2	2-3 Minutes
	Sphinx Pose	20 seconds hold	1	
	Arm Stretch	20 seconds hold each side	1	

Month 3, Week 1-4, Day 1 (Lower Body)

Please scan this QR code for the YouTube Video

Group	Exercise	No. of Reps	No. of Sets	Time Required to Perform
Warm-up	Standing Hip Openers	10	1	5 Minutes
	Air Squats/BW Squats	12	1	
	Hip Flexor Stretch	10 each side	1	
	Quadruped Cat Camel	12	1	
Main workout	Smith Machine Back rack Squats	12	3	15 Minutes
	Landmine Sumo Squats	10	3	
	Landmine Hack Squats	10	3	
	Leg Extension Machine	12	3	
	Seated Calf Raises Machine	12	3	
Cardio	Cycling	NA	NA	8 Minutes
Stretching	Standing Quad Stretch	20 seconds hold each side	1	2-3 Minutes
	Butterfly Stretch	20 seconds hold	1	
	Lying Down Knee Hug	20 seconds hold each side	1	

Month 3, Week 1-4, Day 2 (Upper Body)

Please scan this QR code for the YouTube Video

Group	Exercise	No. of Reps	No. of Sets	Time Required to Perform
Warm-up	3-way Neck Stretch	10 each way	1	5 Minutes
	Shoulder Rotation - Forward & Backward	10 each side	1	
	Smith Machine Incline push-up	10	2	
	Bamboo Stick Shoulder Dislocates	10	1	
Main workout	Barbell Flat Bench Press (start with a small bar initially)	10	3	15 Minutes
	Cable Chest Flys	12	3	
	Shoulder Press Machines	12	3	
	Cable Triceps Pushdown (rope attachment)	12	3	
	Table Top crunches	15	2	
Cardio	Incline Treadmill Walk	NA	NA	8 Minutes
Stretching	Shoulder Stretch	20 seconds hold each side	1	2-3 Minutes
	Wall-assisted Chest Stretch	20 seconds hold	1	
	Triceps Stretch	20 seconds hold each side	1	

Month 3, Week 1-4, Day 3 (Lower Body)

Please scan this QR code for the YouTube Video

Group	Exercise	No. of Reps	No. of Sets	Time Required to Perform
Warm-up	Mountain to Cobra	10	1	5 Minutes
	Bamboo Stick Good Mornings	10	1	
	BW Glute Bridges	12	1	
	Banded Clamshells	10 each side	1	
Main workout	Barbell Hip thrusts	12	3	15 Minutes
	Leg Press (Glute Focused)	12	3	
	Toes Elevated DB Stiff leg Deadlift	10	3	
	Foot Elevated Glute Bridges (Hamstring focused)	10	3	
	Elbow plank to High Plank	30 seconds	2	
Cardio	Cycling	NA	NA	8 Minutes
Stretching	Lying down Glute Stretch	20 seconds hold each side	1	2-3 Minutes
	Hamstring Stretch with Resistance Band	20 seconds hold each side	1	
	Seated Forward bend	20 seconds hold	1	

Month 3, Week 1-4, Day 4 (Upper Body)

Please scan this QR code for the YouTube Video

Group	Exercise	No. of Reps	No. of Sets	Time Required to Perform
Warm-up	Resistance Band Lat pull down	12	1	5 Minutes
	Child's Pose to Cobra	10	1	
	Lying down IYWTO	10 IsYsWsTsOs	1	
	Quadruped T Spine Rotation	10 each side	1	
Main workout	Barbell Upright Rows	12	3	15 Minutes
	Reverse Flys Machine	12	3	
	Cable V Bar Pull Down	12	3	
	Cable Hammer Curl (Rope Attached)	10	3	
	Bamboo Stick Twists	20	2	
Cardio	Incline Treadmill Walk	NA	NA	8 Minutes
Stretching	Twisted Yoga Pose	20 seconds hold	2	2-3 Minutes
	Sphinx Pose	20 seconds hold	1	
	Child's Pose	20 seconds hold	1	

Interactive Reflection And Feedback

We want to hear from you! Reflect on your experience and share your thoughts.

After trying a few of the ready-made gym plans, which one has become your favorite, and why?

_____

_____

_____

_____

How has following a structured plan with warm-ups, targeted exercises, and cool-downs improved your gym experience?

_____

_____

_____

_____

We invite you to submit feedback on the workout plans. Your suggestions will help us improve and tailor plans to meet your needs better.

DETAILED WORKOUT LOG

Keep track of your progress with this comprehensive workout log. Record your workouts, including reps, sets, rest periods, weights carried, and time taken.

Date	Exercise	Weight (lbs/kg)	Sets	Reps
1-Sep-2024	Shoulder Press	10 lbs	3	12

Use this log to monitor your progress, identify areas of improvement, and celebrate your achievements. Remember, consistency is key, and keeping track of your workouts will inspire you and keep your attention on your fitness goals.

After exploring how to maximize your gym experience with focused, effective workouts, the next chapter opens the door to the ongoing adventure of fitness beyond the initial bursts of progress and also about facts about aging bodies experiencing plateaus.

CHAPTER SEVEN
Sustaining Your Fitness Journey

Starting a fitness journey is a great initiative that can lead to a healthier and more satisfying lifestyle. However, the road to reaching fitness goals is often paved with challenges that might challenge your determination. Keeping your motivation high is one of these challenges that might make all the difference in the journey's success.

This chapter will cover the art of staying motivated throughout your fitness journey, providing helpful tips and techniques to help you overcome setbacks and accomplish long-term success. These techniques will help you navigate the ups and downs of your fitness journey, whether you're just getting started or have reached a plateau. They'll also ensure that motivation remains a steadfast companion throughout your life-changing experience.

1. Set Clear and Realistic Goals

It would be like sailing without a compass to embark on a fitness program without a roadmap. The cornerstone of any successful fitness pursuit is the establishment of specific, achievable goals. Instead of vague aims like "getting fit," set specific goals like improving your flexibility, lifting a certain amount of weight, or walking a certain number of steps daily. These specific goals provide direction and meaning to your journey.

Equally important is making sure your goals are achievable. Unrealistic standards can cause frustration and demotivation. Strike a balance between pushing yourself and establishing realistic goals. Long-term goals, like finishing a charity walk or reaching a health milestone, offer a broader perspective, while short-term goals, like Sticking to a regular exercise schedule or learning a new exercise, provide immediate gratification.

You must keep track of your progress. Monitoring your progress regularly shows that you are committed to the task and gives you essential information about what suits you best. Use workout logs, fitness apps, or simple measurements such as loss in inches, clothes fitting better and gain in energy levels to celebrate achievements and recalibrate goals when necessary.

2. Find Your Why

Your fitness journey requires more than physical effort; it also necessitates a profound understanding of your motivations. Reflect on your reasons for wanting to get in shape. Is it to improve your general well-being, increase self-confidence, or set a good example for your family? Connecting with a deeper purpose can significantly enhance your commitment.

Consider how reaching your fitness goals fits your life goals and ideals—discovering your "why" gives your path purpose, which makes the challenges easier to overcome and the victories more satisfying. Many senior women have compelling reasons for embarking on a fitness journey, from overcoming health scares to fulfilling lifelong dreams of being active and vibrant.

3. Mix Up Your Routine

Monotony can be a formidable adversary in your fitness journey. Injecting diversity into your workout program keeps things exciting and enhances overall fitness by working different muscle groups. This book provides diversity, ensuring your fitness journey remains engaging and effective.

Variety can be added with easy changes like trying a new sport, adding interval training, or experimenting with different exercise routines and using different equipment. This maintains the fun and endurance of your workouts. Finding something you love to do turns working out from a chore into a fun experience that improves physical and emotional health.

4. Find a Work out Partner

You don't have to go it alone when starting your fitness journey. Having an exercise partner increases accountability, motivation, and companionship. Challenging exercises can be more fun with a fitness partner, who can also give you the extra motivation you need when you're tired or have self-doubt.

Choose a training partner whose goals for fitness coincide with your own.

A compatible exercise partner, whether a friend, relative, or coworker, can make your fitness journey a shared experience. The dynamic of a supporting relationship is often seen in real-life success stories, demonstrating how encouragement results in perseverance and shared success.

5. Celebrate Small Wins

Your story is a light for others, just as their stories light up your path. Acknowledging and celebrating little accomplishments serves as a powerful motivator. Any progress, no matter how small, is a victory that should be recognized. From improved endurance to gradual weight loss, understanding and appreciating the beneficial changes in your body and overall well-being will help you stay motivated.

Give yourself a meaningful reward to celebrate your accomplishments, such as a favorite meal, a spa day, or new fitness equipment. These benefits reinforce your commitment and give you a sense of accomplishment, transforming challenges into learning experiences.

6. Stay Consistent

Consistency is the basis of a successful fitness journey. You must follow a consistent and reliable exercise routine to see tangible results. Regular exercise improves physical health and creates a routine that helps you stay motivated and dedicated to your goals.

The key to seeing results is to push beyond your comfort zone, not let emotion take over your thinking, and to think from the head, i.e., being disciplined and consistent. There will be days that you will not feel like exercising; pass that moment, get onto a mat, or wear your workout clothes and start your warmup; you will be there!

Planning and commitment are necessary to establish a consistent routine. Sustainability is ensured by creating a fitness regimen that fits your life. Finding a balance that accommodates your personal and professional commitments enhances adherence and lays the foundation for long-term success.

7. Overcome Challenges

Challenges are inevitable on any fitness journey but overcoming them is crucial. Recognize that obstacles like time constraints, plateaus, or unexpected life events are part of the process. Understanding this helps build resilience and mental fortitude.

Address common obstacles with practical strategies, such as finding motivation after a setback, managing time constraints, or navigating physical limitations. Learning from motivational stories of individuals who conquered significant challenges can provide valuable insights and inspire you to stay on course.

8. Seek Professional Guidance

Seeking professional guidance can provide invaluable support on your fitness journey. Fitness professionals, including personal trainers, nutritionists, and coaches, offer specialized knowledge that can accelerate progress and optimize your overall experience.

Choosing the right fitness professional ensures you receive guidance tailored to your goals. Their personalized attention and expertise provide accountability, encouragement, and a structured approach that enhances motivation and results. Professional guidance can be a game-changer whether you're a beginner or aiming for specific outcomes.

By implementing these techniques, you can stay motivated and achieve your fitness goals. Remember, every small step contributes to the larger tapestry of your success. Embrace the challenges, celebrate the victories, and enjoy the journey itself. Your fitness adventure is a testament to your commitment to self-improvement and well-being. Keep moving forward, and the results will undoubtedly follow. Your journey is worth every effort – keep going!

Overcoming Plateaus: Science-Based Tips

Hitting a plateau on your fitness journey can be frustrating, but it's a shared experience you can overcome with some strategic adjustments. Let's dive into science-based strategies to help you push past these plateaus and continue progressing.

1. Make Small Changes in Nutrition

What you eat is very important to your fitness progress. If you've hit a plateau, it might be time to tweak your diet. Consider reducing or adding a few calories to see how your body responds. Sometimes, a slight caloric deficit or surplus can reignite your metabolism. Focus on balanced meals rich in complex carbs, healthy fats, and protein to sustain your workouts and recovery.

2. Increase Reps or Sets

If your current workout routine has become too easy, it's a sign that your body has adapted. Increasing the number of reps or sets can add to the challenge you need to break through a plateau. For instance, if you're doing ten reps of a particular exercise, try increasing it to 12 or 15. This added volume can stimulate muscle growth and strength gain.

3. Boost Resistance

Gradually increasing the resistance of your dumbbells or resistance bands can also help you overcome a plateau. If you've been lifting the same weight for a while, your muscles have likely adapted. Challenge them by moving up to a heavier weight. Even small increments can make a big difference in your progress.

4. Add More Steps

Increasing your daily step count is another effective way to break through a plateau. Aim to add an extra 1,000 steps to your daily total. This can be as simple as taking a brisk walk in the evening or incorporating more movement into your day, like using the stairs rather than the elevator or parking far away from your destination.

5. Stay Hydrated and Get Enough Rest

Hydration and rest are often overlooked but are crucial for overcoming plateaus. Dehydration can hinder your performance, and lack of sleep can affect your recovery and energy levels. Ensure you drink enough water throughout the day and get 7-8 hours of sleep each night.

6. Mix Up Your Routine

Sometimes, your body needs a new challenge. Try incorporating different kinds of exercises into your routine. If you typically do strength training, add cardio or flexibility workouts like yoga or Pilates. This variety can shock your muscles and prevent boredom.

7. Track Your Progress

Keeping a workout journal can help you identify patterns and make informed adjustments. Note your exercises, reps, sets, weights, and how you feel during and after workouts. This data can reveal what changes are most effective in overcoming your plateau.

8. Consult a Professional

If you're having trouble breaking through a plateau despite your best efforts, consider consulting a fitness professional or a nutritionist. They can offer personalized advice and modifications based on your needs and goals.

Remember, hitting plateaus is a common occurrence on any fitness journey. By making these small, science-based changes, you can push past them and continue making progress. Stay consistent, listen to your body, and keep challenging yourself. You've got this!

Share Your Journey

Tag and Post Your Transformation

We would love to see your progress and hear your thoughts! Tag this book and share your transformation or review on social media. Your journey can inspire and motivate others just beginning or continuing their fitness journey. Don't forget to use the hashtag #StrengthTrainingOver50 to connect with a community of like-minded women.

What's Your Favorite "At Home" Exercise?

We all have that one exercise we look forward to and rely on in our routines. What's yours? Share your favorite at-home exercise that has become a staple in your routine. Whether it's a go-to strength training move, a relaxing stretch, or a fun cardio burst, your favorites can inspire others to diversify their workouts and find new joy in fitness.

The real adventure is just beginning as we close this chapter of your journey within these pages. Don't wait for a perfect moment; make this moment perfect by taking your first step today. Let your fitness journey be a testament to the power of starting now, where every day brings you closer to your goals. Ready, set, let's move!

Conclusion

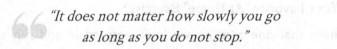

> *"It does not matter how slowly you go
> as long as you do not stop."*
> — Confucius

Congratulations on taking this empowering journey towards strength and well-being! You've taken a bold step by embracing strength training, proving that age is no barrier to becoming stronger, healthier, and more confident.

As you've seen throughout this book, strength training offers numerous benefits, from improving bone density and muscle mass to boosting your metabolism and overall quality of life. By committing to a consistent strength training routine, you are investing in your future health and independence.

Remember, it's not just about the physical strength you gain but also the mental resilience you build along the way. Each workout is a testament to your dedication and determination. Celebrate every small victory, whether lifting a heavier weight, feeling more energetic, or simply enjoying a better night's sleep.

Stay consistent and listen to your body. It's important to push yourself, but equally important to rest and recover. Adjust your routine as needed and seek support from fitness communities, trainers, or workout partners who can keep you motivated and accountable.

You are part of a growing community of strong, vibrant women over 50 who are redefining what it means to age. By prioritizing your health and well-being, you set an inspiring example for others and prove that it's never too late to start.

Thank you for allowing me to be a part of your strength training journey. Keep lifting, moving, and, most importantly, believing in your incredible potential.

References

Artyshchuk, O. (2022, March 30). Fiber and protein: Why a high protein high fiber diet will change your life - MyCHN Community Health Network. MyCHN Community Health Network. https://mychn.org/fiber-and-protein/

Best, N. (n.d.). How to calculate BMR and TDEE and why you should. Natures Best. https://www.naturesbest.co.uk/sports-articles/how-to-calculate-bmr-and-tdee-and-why-you-should/

Better aging: 10 tips for Changing your Mindset. (2024, April 26). https://www.baystatehealth.org/articles/10-tips-for-aging-well

Bhg-Admin. (2024, May 29). Achievable senior fitness goals for the New Year - Bethesda Health Group. Bethesda Health Group. https://bethesdahealth.org/blog/2022/01/14/achievable-senior-fitness-goals-for-2022/#:~:text=Your%20fitness%20goals%20should%20include,assess%20where%20you%20are%20physically.

Breeding, B. (2023, August 3). Positive Aging: Changing your mindset about growing older | MyLifeSite. myLifeSite. https://mylifesite.net/blog/post/positive-aging-changing-mindset-gRowing-older/

Castro-Sloboda, G. (2022, December 7). Knowing your BMR can improve your chances of losing weight and more. CNET. https://www.cnet.com/health/fitness/your-basal-metabolic-rate-bmr-is-the-key-to-losing-weight-or-gaining-muscle/

Comfort Keepers. (n.d.). Elements of a good exercise program for older adults. https://www.comfortkeepers.com/offices/minnesota/osseo/resources/resources/elements-of-a-good-exercise-program-for-older-adults/

Cpt, K. D. M. R. (2021, September 20). The definitive guide to healthy eating in your 50s and 60s. Healthline.

https://www.healthline.com/nutrition/healthy-eating-50s-60s#nutrients-foods

Dogra, T. (2023, September 26). 5 Strategies for sustaining motivation in your fitness journey | TheHealthSite.com. TheHealthSite. https://www.thehealthsite.com/fitness/fitness-workouts-fitness/5-strategies-for-sustaining-motivation-in-your-fitness-journey-1014159/

Donvito, T. (2024, April 26). Your body at 50 - Keck Medicine of USC. Keck Medicine of USC. https://hie.keckmedicine.org/blog/your-body-at-50/

Emma. (2023, June 20). Why is strength training important for menopause? https://www.bupa.co.uk/newsroom/ourviews/strength-training-menopause

Erin. (2024, June 23). Healthy habits for seniors' daily routine. Centers Health Care. https://centershealthcare.com/media/four-healthy-habits-for-seniors-to-add-to-their-daily-routine/

Five essential elements of elderly exercise. (n.d.). University of Iowa Health Care. https://uihc.org/health-topics/five-essential-elements-elderly-exercise

Friends Healthcare. (2024, January 31). Embracing the Golden Years: A Guide to Celebrating Aging for Seniors | Friends Care Community. Friends Care Community. https://friendshealthcare.org/2023/07/20/embracing-the-golden-years-a-guide-to-celebrating-aging-for-seniors/

Garone, S. (2021, September 30). The definitive guide to adapt your fitness routine for every phase of life. Healthline. https://www.healthline.com/health/the-definitive-guide-to-adapting-your-fitness-routine-for-every-phase-of-life#safety

Getting SMART about goal setting for seniors. (2022, December 30). https://www.hebrewseniorlife.org/blog/getting-smart-about-goal-setting-seniors

How to Change your mindset and promote positive aging | Resort Lifestyle Communities | Resort Lifestyle Communities. (n.d.). Resort Lifestyle Communities. https://rlcommunities.com/blog/how-to-change-your-mindset-and-promote-positive-aging/

Howard, B. (2012, September 21). What to Expect in your 50s. AARP. https://www.aarp.org/health/healthy-living/info-09-2012/what-to-expect-in-your-50s.html

Hrustic, A., Matthews, M., & Blumberg, P. O. (2024, June 26). 15 ways to break through a weight loss plateau. Men's Health. https://www.menshealth.com/weight-loss/a19537316/weight-loss-plateau/

Human Kinetics. (n.d.). Strength training during menopause offers multiple benefits. https://us.humankinetics.com/blogs/excerpt/strength-training-during-menopause-offers-multiple-benefits

Keegan, D. (2022, February 16). Tips to sustain your fitness journey. Temple Gym Varsity Lakes. https://www.templegym.com.au/tips-to-sustain-your-fitness-journey/

LCMC Health. (2021, December 15). 6 tips for exercising safely as an older adult. https://www.lcmchealth.org/touro/blog/2021/december/6-tips-for-exercising-safely-as-an-older-adult/

Pajer, N. (2024, January 10). 9 nutrients you need more of as you get older. AARP. https://www.aarp.org/health/healthy-living/info-2023/essential-nutrients-for-healthy-aging.html

Phelps, N. (2019, March 29). What is BMR and TDEE + How to use them to lose weight. Chomps. https://chomps.com/blogs/nutrition-sustainability-news/what-is-bmr-tdee

Richardson, M. (2024, February 13). Exercise to build muscle: A Natural Rememdy for Menopause symptoms. Harrison Healthcare. https://harrisonhealthcare.ca/exercise-muscle-build-menopause/

Seo, R. D. (n.d.). » The role of exercise in managing Menopause Symptoms. https://www.menopausecentre.com.au/information-centre/articles/the-role-of-exercise-in-managing-menopause-symptoms/#:~:text=Recommended%20exercises%20for%20menopausal%20women&text=Strength%20training%3A%20this%20is%20one,resistance%20training%2C%20or%20bodyweight%20exercises.

Setting SMART goals to improve senior fitness. (2024, January 23). https://www.alert-1.com/blog/general/setting-smart-goals-to-improve-senior-fitness

Sirois, L. (2023, September 6). Nutrition for Seniors: Protein and fiber. Visavie. https://visavie.com/en/nutrition-for-seniors-protein-and-fiber

Spritzler, F. (2024, February 26). 12 simple ways to break through a weight loss plateau. Healthline. https://www.healthline.com/nutrition/weight-loss-plateau#track-your-foods

SR, V. (2022, August 8). What to know about core exercises for Seniors. WebMD. https://www.webmd.com/fitness-exercise/what-to-know-about-core-exercises-for-seniors

St. Andrew's Resources for Senior System. (2023, October 18). Cardio Exercises for Seniors—Benefits & best Aerobic activities. St. Andrew's. https://standrews1.com/blog/cardio-exercises-for-seniors/

Staying motivated to exercise: tips for older adults. (2020, April 3). National Institute on Aging. https://www.nia.nih.gov/health/exercise-and-physical-activity/staying-motivated-exercise-tips-older-adults

Stefanacci, R. G. (2024, April 10). Changes in the body with aging. MSD Manual Consumer Version. https://www.msdmanuals.com/home/older-people%E2%80%99s-health-issues/the-aging-body/changes-in-the-body-with-aging#Ears_v8967919

The benefits of cardio exercise for seniors. (n.d.). https://www.villageatwoodsedge.com/post/the-benefits-of-cardio-exercise-for-seniors

The Best Exercise Warmup For Seniors - Physio Ed. (2024, July 22). Physioed. https://physioed.com/exercise-warmup-for-seniors/

The Goodman Group. (n.d.). Safety considerations for seniors starting a new exercise program. https://blog.thegoodmangroup.com/safety-considerations-for-seniors-starting-a-new-exercise-program

Trotta, R. (2023, January 2). How protein and fiber will change your body. Rachel Trotta. https://racheltrotta.com/fitness/protein-and-fiber-will-change-your-body/

Velarde, J. (2023, August 8). Aging gracefully: the power of positive thinking. Senior Friendship Centers. https://friendshipcenters.org/aging-gracefully-the-power-of-positive-thinking/#:~:text=This%20simple%20act%20can%20shift,walking%2C%20yoga%2C%20or%20dancing.

What to expect in your 50s. (n.d.). WebMD. https://www.webmd.com/healthy-aging/ss/slideshow-what-to-expect-in-your-50s